Robert D. Rubens

Editor

The management of bone metastases and hypercalcaemia by osteoclast inhibition

An international symposium held during the
5th European Conference on Clinical Oncology
(ECCO 5), London, September 1989

D1302385

Hogrefe & Huber Publishers
Toronto · Lewiston N.Y. · Bern · Göttingen · Stuttgart

© Copyright 1990 by Hans Huber Publishers

12–14 Bruce Park Ave.
Toronto, Ontario M4P 2S3

P.O. Box 51
Lewiston, N.Y. 14092

Printed in Switzerland

ISBN 0–88937–047–8
Hogrefe & Huber Publishers · Toronto · Lewiston N.Y. · Bern · Göttingen · Stuttgart
ISBN 3–456–81922–6
Hogrefe & Huber Publishers · Bern · Göttingen · Stuttgart · Toronto · Lewiston N.Y.

Contents

5

Participants

Chairman

R. D. RUBENS, ICRF Clinical Oncology Unit, Guy's Hospital, London SE1 9RT, UK

Contributors

O. L. M. BIJVOET, Department of Clinical Endocrinology and Metabolism, University Hospital, Rijsburgerweg 10, 2333 AA Leiden, The Netherlands

P. BURCKHARDT, Department of Internal Medicine, Centre Hospitalier Universitaire Vaudois, CH-1011 Lausanne, Switzerland

N. W. CLARKE, Department of Surgery, Withington Hospital, Nell Lane, West Didsbury, Manchester M20 8LR, UK

R. E. COLEMAN, Department of Clinical Oncology, Western General Hospital, Crewe Road, Edinburgh EH4 2XU, UK

D. J. DODWELL, Department of Medical Oncology, Christie Hospital, Wilmslow Road, Withington, Manchester M20 9BX, UK

A. L. HARRIS, ICRF Clinical Oncology Unit, Churchill Hospital, Headington, Oxford OX3 7LJ, UK

S. LEYVRAZ, Departement d'Oncologie Universitaire et Institut Ludwig, Centre Hospitalier Universitaire Vaudois, CH-1011 Lausanne, Switzerland

A. LIPTON, Division of Medical Oncology, Milton S. Hershey Medical Center, PO Box 850, Hershey, Pennsylvania 17033, USA

H. T. MOURIDSEN, Department of Oncology, Finsen Institute, 49 Strandboulevarden, DK-2100 Copenhagen, Denmark

S. R. NUSSBAUM, Endocrine Unit, Massachusetts General Hospital and Harvard Medical School, Boston, Massachusetts 02114, USA

S. H. RALSTON, Rheumatic Diseases Unit, Northern General Hospital, Ferry Road, Edinburgh EH5 2DQ, UK

P. RITCH, Hematology/Oncology Section, Medical College of Wisconsin, 8700 W Wisconsin Avenue, Milwaukee, Wisconsin 53226, USA

F. WINGEN, Institute of Toxicology and Chemotherapy, German Cancer Research Centre, D-6900 Heidelberg, Federal Republic of Germany

7

Preface

The clinical problems of hypercalcaemia and bone metastases

Bone metastases in patients with cancer cause extensive morbidity, much of it attributable to hypercalcaemia. Yet relatively little clinical research has been applied to these common problems in the past. Approaches to treatment have often been empirical and non-specific, with bone metastases sometimes appearing to respond poorly to endocrine and cytotoxic therapy when compared with metastases in other tissues. Undoubtedly, these difficulties have been due, at least in part, to the imprecise methods available for assessing the response of bony lesions to treatment. While progress has been made in identifying biochemical indices as early predictors of response, plain radiography remains the standard method of assessment. Although isotope scanning provides a sensitive method for detecting lesions, it is of little value for monitoring response.

Bone metastases are a major problem in breast cancer. In a series of 587 deaths from breast cancer (COLEMAN and RUBENS, 1987a), an antemortem diagnosis of bone metastases was made in over two-thirds of the patients (Table I); the high incidence of bone metastasis as the first site of distant relapse is shown in Table II. If metastatic disease remains confined to the skeleton, survival can

Table I. Bone metastases in breast cancer. Antemortem diagnosis of metastases in 587 deaths from breast cancer (Guy's Hospital Breast Unit, 1979–84).

Bone	69%
Lung	27%
Liver	27%

Table II. Incidence of bone metastases as first site of distant relapse in 2240 breast cancer patients (Guy's Hospital Breast Unit, 1979–84).

Overall	8%
Those with any recurrence	24%
Those with distant metastases	47%

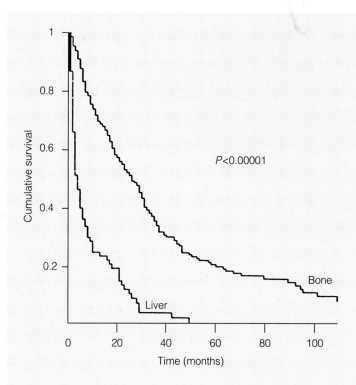

Fig.1. Pattern of survival following first relapse: cases with metastatic disease confined to the skeleton ($n = 253$) compared to those with liver metastases ($n = 72$).

Table III. Breast cancer complications. Frequency after first relapse in bone among 498 breast cancer patients (Guy's Hospital Breast Unit, 1979–84).

Hypercalcaemia	17%
Pathological fracture	16%
Spinal cord compression	3%

however be prolonged for a median of 24 months, with 20% of patients alive at five years, compared to a median survival of only three months among patients with liver metastases (Fig. 1).

The relatively long survival of many patients with skeletal metastases is associated with a wide spectrum of morbidity including pain, fracture, bone-marrow suppression, neurological impairment, and hypercalcaemia (Table III). Growing recognition of hypercalcaemia has particularly focused attention on the crucial importance of the osteoclast as a mediator of neoplastic damage in bone, leading us to realise the therapeutic potential for inhibitors of these cells. Osteoclast inhibition can be effectively achieved by the bisphosphonates, and pamidronate has become the agent of choice for treating hypercalcaemia (COLEMAN and RUBENS, 1987b). The recent demonstration that it can actually reverse osteolysis, enabling recalcification of bone to take place, is of major therapeutic significance (COLEMAN et al, 1988).

This symposium, held during the 5th European Conference on Clinical Oncology in London, presented much new information on the role of pamidronate and other bisphosphonates in the treatment of patients with hypercalcaemia and bone metastases. Publication of this report is designed to make that information more widely available with a minimum of delay.

Robert D. Rubens

References

COLEMAN, R.E. and RUBENS, R.D. (1987a) The clinical course of bone metastases from breast cancer. *Br. J. Cancer 55*, 61–66.

COLEMAN, R.E. and RUBENS, R.D. (1987b) 3(amino-1,1-hydroxypropylidene) bisphosphonate (APD) for hypercalcaemia of breast cancer. *Br. J. Cancer 56*, 465–469.

COLEMAN, R.E., WOLL, P.J., MILES, M. et al (1988) Treatment of bone metastases from breast cancer with 3(amino-1-hydroxypropylidene)-1,1-bisphosphonate (APD). *Br. J. Cancer 58*, 621–625.

Pamidronate (APD) in cancer therapy – the pharmacological background

O. L. M. Bijvoet

Professor of Medicine and Endocrinology, University Hospital, Leiden,
The Netherlands

Summary

Pamidronate (APD) is effective in the therapy of acute and chronic hypercalcaemia associated with bone metastases. When given intravenously in high doses over a short period it prevents bone resorption by inhibiting osteoclast activity, thereby lessening bone pain and hypercalcaemia. Long-term, low-dose oral treatment with pamidronate partially prevents pathological bone resorption, leading to decreased morbidity.

The cycle of cellular activity in bone is described with special reference to interactions between different bone cells. Bisphosphonates prevent osteoclasts from recognising bone as such and thus prevent new cycles of bone resorption in several conditions, including bone metastases, Paget's disease and osteoporosis. Bisphosphonates also indirectly reduce the rate of new bone formation and remodelling: caution is therefore needed when administering high doses since their long-term use may increase the incidence of fractures. When high doses are needed initially, they should be reduced in patients requiring longer term treatment.

Bisphosphonates do not appear to have any cumulative effect. The risk of fractures is not significantly increased by long-term bisphosphonate therapy at low dosage. Preventive therapy may therefore be indicated in patients with breast cancer likely to metastasise to bone and perhaps in postmenopausal osteoporosis and other conditions.

Introduction

Bisphosphonates all have a characteristic primary P–C–P structure which enables them to adhere to crystal surfaces. In physical chemistry, they alter the energy-dependent interactions between the crystal phase and the surrounding phase and thus change their properties, including crystal growth and dissolution (FRANCIS, 1983).

In the body too, the bisphosphonates have a high affinity for the crystal surfaces in mineralised matrix of bone. When present on this surface they inhibit its resorption by osteoclasts (FLEISCH, 1983). The potency and specificity of the bisphosphonates for the latter largely depend on their secondary structure, which can take various forms (Fig. 1) (BOONEKAMP et al, 1986, 1987). After longer periods of time, by virtue of the particular role of osteoclast resorption in the dynamics of the bone remodelling process, the bisphospho-

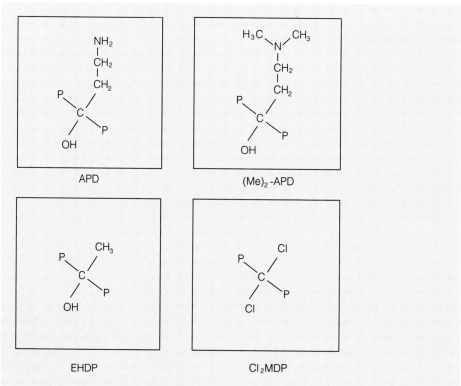

Fig. 1. Structure of four bisphosphonates: pamidronate (APD), dimethyl pamidronate ([Me]₂-APD), etidronate (EHDP) and clodronate (Cl₂MDP).

nates may alter functional characteristics of bone that are not immediately predictable from their short-term action. Consequently, bisphosphonates can be applied as pharmacological tools in two quite different settings:

- One characteristically exploits the properties of the drug for short-term, therapeutic goals, which commonly involve the suppression of undesirable, excessive bone resorption – as in the treatment of hypercalcaemia of malignancy or the suppression of resorption due to the presence of malignant cells.
- The other, long-term setting is exploited in secondary prevention of bone disease through alteration of bone remodelling characteristics and involves the induction of reduced vulnerability for pathological processes that tend to induce excessive bone breakdown. An example is the use of bisphosphonates as supportive treatment to obtain reduction of future morbidity in breast cancer patients with metastatic bone disease.

Dose requirements and administration schedules may be quite different for the two types of application. Whereas the efficacy and safety of a bisphosphonate in the short-term setting may be closely related to its potency and specificity *in*

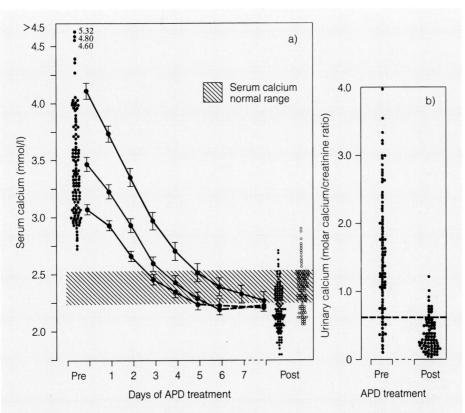

Fig. 2. (a) Serum calcium before and after treatment with pamidronate in 132 patients with tumour-induced hypercalcaemia. *Solid circles* indicate total serum calcium values, and *open circles* indicate calcium values after correction for serum albumin. The normal range is indicated by the *shaded area*. The curves represent averages of serum calcium (mean ± s.e. mean) during treatment after division into three groups according to pretreatment serum calcium level (<3.25, $n = 61$; >3.75, $n = 25$; the remainder, $n = 46$). Note that the total amount of pamidronate given until normalisation increases with the pretreatment serum calcium level. (b) Molar urinary calcium/creatinine ratio in the same patients before and after treatment. The *broken line* is the upper limit of normal (data after Harinck et al, 1987b).

vitro, the predicted efficacy in the long-term setting depends rather on pharmacokinetic and in particular on pharmacodynamic considerations.

The first half of this symposium contains detailed papers on the therapeutic value of pamidronate (APD) for lowering blood calcium levels in hypercalcaemia of malignancy. Figure 2 shows typical results obtained in a large group of hypercalcaemic patients given 15 mg daily. Nearly all became normocalcaemic within 3–5 days, evidently due to reduction in bone resorption (a), followed by a decrease in urinary calcium excretion (b).

The second half of the symposium is concerned with pamidronate treatment of the metastatic bone disease that often underlies hypercalcaemia in cancer

15

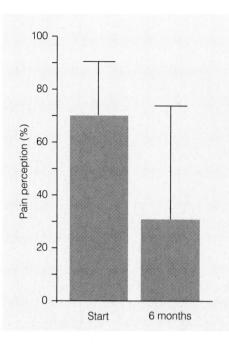

Fig. 3. Effect of pamidronate (30 mg i.v. weekly for four weeks, fortnightly thereafter) in reducing pain associated with metastatic bone disease in 16 patients, as measured by linear analogue scale (data after MORTON et al, 1988).

Table I. Interruption of bone resorption – complete or partial.

Complete

High dose; short-term; usually intravenous; *reduces* pain (from bone metastases) and possibly sclerosis; anti-tumour effect; possible anti-inflammatory effect

Partial

Low dose; long-term; usually oral; *prevents* increased size and number of metastases; reduces access to new matrix

patients. This has been shown to improve X-ray appearances (MORTON et al, 1988) and to reduce pain in such patients (Fig. 3). There is also evidence, not detailed at this symposium, that pamidronate may be effective in preventing further skeletal morbidity due to bone metastases. Figure 4 shows the rising incidence of complications due to metastatic bone disease in 85 breast cancer patients not treated with pamidronate, compared with the same number given low doses of pamidronate orally. The cumulative reduction in complications reaches approximately 50%.

Taking this evidence together, pamidronate has unquestionably been shown to possess potent therapeutic or preventive properties in acute and chronic conditions associated with bone metastases. The pharmacological background to these actions may be considered in two distinct therapeutic categories (Table I).

Approaches to therapy

In the treatment of acute conditions, 'complete' interruption of pathological bone resorption is obtained by giving a large dose of pamidronate over a short period, normally by intravenous infusion. This appears to prevent osteoclasts from identifying bone as a target tissue and thus inhibits their activity – with consequent reduction in bone pain and hypercalcaemia. The reduction of bone pain and eventual induction of sclerosis, which have been observed in active bone metastases, should not necessarily be considered an effect of the drug on the tumour itself. It is quite possible that local excessive osteoclastic bone resorption is accompanied by secondary inflammatory phenomena. This would for instance explain the presence of local oedema and signs of inflammation, associated with pain, often observed in Paget's disease (FRIJLINK et al, 1979; HARINCK et al, 1987a). Interruption of osteoclastic resorption with calcitonin or bisphosphonates is rapidly followed by reduction of local hyperaemia, pain, and even sclerosis of lytic bone lesions. It is not impossible that a similar cycle of events occurs in metastatic breast cancer, since the pain starts when the periosteum begins to be elevated, perhaps partly by inflammatory oedema. Some anti-inflammatory effect of pamidronate, mediated via osteoclast inhibition, cannot be ruled out.

The second therapeutic option is 'partial' interruption of bone resorption during long-term preventive treatment with smaller doses of pamidronate, which may be given orally. This will not produce any therapeutic effect demonstrable in individual patients but, as noted above (see also Fig. 4), comparison of groups may reveal a 50% decrease in morbidity among patients receiving pamidronate.

Mechanisms of action

How are these changes brought about? Figure 5 portrays the cyclic nature of bone as an ecosystem in which there are two main populations of fixed and mobile cells. *Fixed mesenchymal stem cells* form the lining cells of bone and are the ancestors of osteoblasts and also of the fibroblasts in bone and of the supporting cells in vessel walls. *Mobile cells* are derived from haematopoetic stem cells and consist of monocytes, macrophages, lymphocytes, and osteoclasts – which may be likened to tissue macrophages of bone. All these cells interact, with osteoblasts responsible for maintaining bone formation, balancing osteoclast activity which causes bone resorption (NIJWEIDE, 1986). Their mechanisms of interaction are not yet fully understood, but factors coming from osteoclasts or liberated from bone appear to be essential in inducing osteoblast precursors to become osteoblasts, which can be seen as specialised fibroblasts. Equally, osteoclasts cannot function without osteoblasts, which not only produce factors that induce proliferation of osteoclast precursors, but also factors that adhere to the bone surface and alter it in such a way that the osteoclast precursors can recognise it. Without this recognition, it is impossible for an osteoclast precursor to differentiate into a mature osteoclast able to break down bone (BARON et al, 1984; HORTON, 1988; RAISZ, 1988). Formation of osteoclast precursors and their development into osteoclasts can also be induced by the macrophage/lymphocyte system, and tumours may activate this

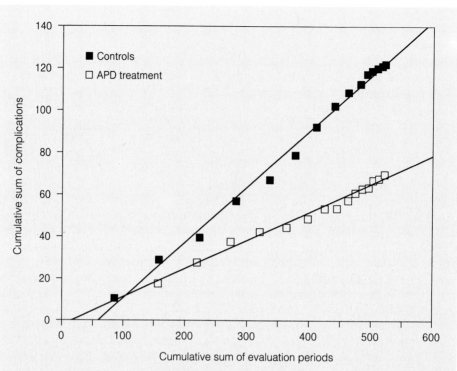

Fig. 4. Cumulative complications due to metastatic bone disease in two groups of 85 breast cancer patients, over subsequent three-monthly observation periods, treated with 300 mg oral pamidronate daily *(open squares)* and not treated *(closed squares)*. The slope of the lines represents the three-monthly incidence in each group (data after VAN HOLTEN-VERZANTVOORT, 1990; VAN HOLTEN-VERZANTVOORT et al, 1987).

pathway. Nevertheless, it would be impossible for osteoclasts to start breaking down bone without the presence of an osteoblast-derived factor – as further discussed below.

Views on the mechanism by which the inhibitory effect of bisphosphonates on osteoclastic bone resorption is achieved, vary widely. These views can be classified in three groups:

1. Ingested bisphosphonate may be toxic for the resorbing osteoclast (BOONE-KAMP et al, 1986; FLANAGAN and CHAMBERS, 1989; REITSMA et al, 1982). The phenomenon has been seen *in vitro,* particularly with clodronate. For two reasons this may not be the explanation for *in vivo* activity. One is that the relative molar potency of bisphosphonates with respect to this property does not reflect their relative potencies as resorption inhibitors *in vivo;* the second is that neither whole animal nor clinical studies have shown similar toxic changes in osteoclasts. The studies do however show that some bisphosphonates may be more toxic than others, a phenomenon that could be considered in relation to clinical acceptability.

2. Surface-bound bisphosphonate may maintain a concentration gradient of bisphosphonate, near the bone surface, sufficiently large to let bisphospho-

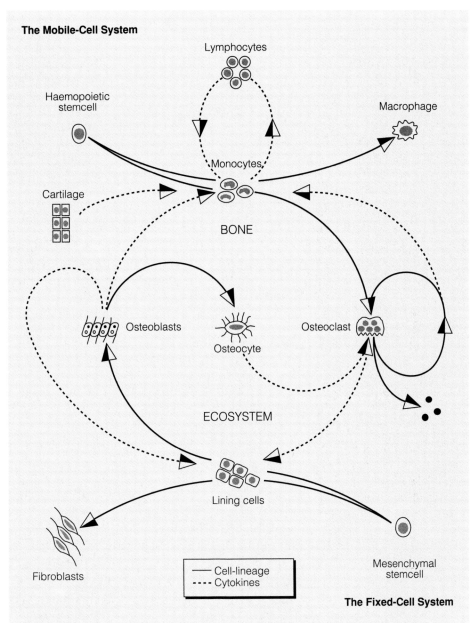

The Mobile-Cell System

Lymphocytes

Haemopoietic
stemcell

Macrophage

Monocytes

Cartilage

BONE

Osteoblasts

Osteocyte

Osteoclast

ECOSYSTEM

Lining cells

Cell-lineage
Cytokines

Fibroblasts

Mesenchymal
stemcell

The Fixed-Cell System

Fig. 5. The 'bone ecosystem'. Conceptual image of cell lineage *(curves)* and cell-cell interaction *(interrupted curves)* between and in the two major cell families of bone.

nates have a direct influence on osteoclast progenitor cells or on other cell
systems that are operative in initiating bone resorption (BIJVOET et al, 1980;
CECCHINI et al, 1987; LERNER and LARSSON, 1987). Isolated cells will alter a
variety of metabolic properties and even the ability to proliferate in the
presence of quite low doses of bisphosphonates; but other effects, like those on   19

proliferation of osteoclast precursors, vary according to the *in vivo* potency of the bisphosphonate. We now consider it unlikely that this represents the mechanism of action. *In vivo* inhibition of resorption is not associated with a reduction in osteoclasts or osteoclast precursors, but – depending on the circumstance – with an increase in osteoclast-like cells. Futhermore, subsequent exposure of a bisphosphonate-pretreated bone explant to resorbing cells results in less resorption, without bisphosphonate in the medium (BOONEKAMP et al, 1986, 1987; LÖWIK et al, 1988). The molar potency of the bisphosphonate is the same, whether used for pretreatment or only added during exposure to osteoclasts. Although bisphosphonates do 'desorb' from bone it is unlikely that they can maintain a sufficiently high bisphosphonate concentration in the bone environment for this mechanism to be relevant. But, again, the studies show that circulating bisphosphonates have surprisingly large effects on cell metabolism. It would be wise to avoid high circulating concentrations during treatment.

3. Osteoclastic bone resorption may require a signal from matrix-bound cytokines to osteoclast precursors in order to activate their resorptive potential (BOONEKAMP et al, 1986, 1987; LÖWIK et al, 1988; HUGHES et al, 1989). Osteoclast precursors accede to the bone surface through chemo-attraction and subsequently, after coming into contact with osteoblast-derived cytokines, bind to the calcified matrix, which activates their resorptive potency (BARON et al, 1984; HORTON, 1988; RAISZ, 1988). *In vitro* model systems, consisting of bone explants that have been prepared in such a way that their resorption depends on prior activation by the bone matrix of osteoclast precursors, have been used to show that pretreatment of those explants with bisphosphonate does inhibit the ability of the explant to induce differentiation of the osteoclast precursor into a mature resorbing osteoclast. Subsequent resorption is prevented to a degree that depends on the bisphosphonate concentration to which the explants had been exposed. The relative molar potencies of bisphosphonates in these systems do closely reflect their inhibitor potential *in vivo* (BOONEKAMP et al, 1986, 1987; LÖWIK et al, 1988). In those systems, inhibition depends soley on matrix-bound bisphosphonate and does not require the presence of bisphosphonate in the medium. Within the identical experiment, tissue that has calcified after exposure to the drug, and is therefore not covered with bisphosphonate, retains the potential to be resorbed. It is therefore unlikely that surface-bound and not circulating bisphosphonate is responsible for the inhibitor action. For the various reasons that have been mentioned, this third mechanism is the most likely to be responsible for the inhibitory effect of the bisphosphonates *in vivo*. Thus bisphosphonates appear to prevent osteoclastic resorption, rather than inhibit it.

If bisphosphonates do preclude rather than inhibit osteoclastic resorption, their great clinical efficacy has to reflect a large dependency of normal resorption on continuous generation of new osteoclasts. Data on osteoclast turnover are not incompatible with the possibility that these cells depend on continued fusion with new precursors to replace loss of nuclear material, the replacement rate of the latter being quite rapid, in the order of five days (BARON et al, 1984; JAWORSKI et al, 1981). It is now accepted that maintenance of the viability of bone as a tissue depends on close cyclic interaction of the various cell systems present within this organ, an interaction mediated through local messenger molecules, the cytokines. Activation of new osteoclasts precursors, their accession to bone under chemotactic influence, and their differentiation upon contact with the bone acting as a solid cytokine (the bisphosphonate-sensitive process) are all modulated or mediated by cytokines originating from osteoblasts (RAISZ, 1988). Even the stimulation of bone resorption by parathyroid hormone is mediated through the osteoblast.

The inhibitory action *in vivo* is therefore analogous to the way bisphosphonates act in pure crystal systems – by altering surface properties (BOONEKAMP et al, 1987; LÖWIK et al, 1988). The importance of surface binding also has consequences for the interpretation of pharmacokinetic studies. Bone-surface bound bisphosphonate should be considered as a compartment distinct from the remainder of the bisphosphonate taken up into the bone. Surface-bound bisphosphonate could theoretically disappear by three mechanisms: physico-chemical 'desorption', removal by resorbing osteoclasts, and incorporation in the bone mass during osteoblastic bone formation. Since the last two may contribute considerably to the turnover of surface-bound bisphosphonate, the biological activity in low bone-turnover states may be more prolonged than in high remodelling states. Moreover, inhibition of the rate of bone remodelling would lead to a reduction in the rate of disappearance of surface-bound bisphosphonate. Whatever the reason, the disappearance of the pharmacological effect of a given bisphosphonate dose may be much faster than the overall disappearance of bisphosphonate from bone.

Effects on bone

Returning to the dynamic cycle of cellular activity in bone (Fig. 5), osteoclast nuclei have a survival time of only five days, whereas osteoblasts live for three to six months. Therefore osteoblastic laying down of new bone continues long after osteoclastic bone resorption has been inhibited. This is clearly demonstrated by hydroxyproline excretion falling within days of starting bisphosphonate therapy, reflecting the decline in bone resorption, to be followed after a long delay by a decline in bone formation, as evidenced by the fall in alkaline phosphatase (Fig. 6). Clearly long-term bisphosphonates in high dosage do ultimately reduce bone turnover as a whole. This could be potentially dangerous.

When bone formation is measured by the percentage of surface labelled with tetracycline, the incidence of fractures has been shown to rise (in dogs) as new bone formation declines under the influence of bisphosphonates. This has been demonstrated for clodronate and etidronate, and is likely to be equally true of pamidronate (FLORA, 1981). Caution is therefore required about high-dosage, long-term therapy with any of these compounds – particularly as bisphosphonates have a long residence time in bone, with a five-year half-life.

Do these observations mean that patients on long-term bisphosphonate treatment will eventually get spontaneous fractures? Studies in young rats have shown that the rate and degree of suppression of bone resorption – as measured by reduced hydroxyproline excretion – are both dose dependent (Fig. 7), 21

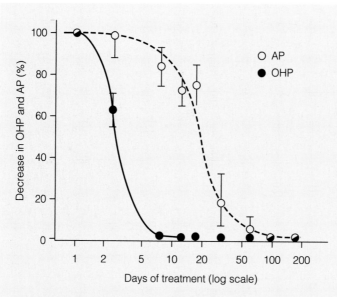

Fig. 6. Urinary hydroxyproline (OHP) excretion rate *(closed circles; line)* and serum alkaline phosphatase (AP) activity *(open circles; interrupted line)* before and during treatment with pamidronate in patients with Paget's disease. Values are expressed as percentage of the initial excess above the upper limit of the normal range. Note that the suppression of excessive bone resorption, reflected in the normalisation of OHP, precedes the normalisation of bone formation, measured as AP, by three months (after FRIJLINK et al, 1979).

and that the degree of suppression remains stable despite continued administration. This suggests that the level of suppression can be adjusted by changes in dosage. In humans given lower doses of pamidronate orally over several years for osteoporosis (150 mg oral ®Aredia per day), we found a stable 20% reduction of bone turnover (Fig. 8) (unpublished). This study revealed no evidence of a cumulative effect, which is extremely important in long-term therapy where too high a dose should be avoided. The evidence that bisphosphonates have a long half-life and therefore tend to cumulate in bone, and the evidence that the biological effect does not cumulate, are not necessarily in contradiction. The pharmacokinetic studies that measure total bone bisphosphonate do not necessarily measure the *biologically active* bisphosphonate. If, as suggested, the biologically active bisphosphonate is contained in a separate, discrete, surface compartment of bone, it is conceivable that that compartment reaches equilibrium between gain of new material through adsorption and loss through desorption, resorption and osteoblastic burial, while the process of burial continues to contribute to the inactive, deep-bone bisphosphonate. It is evident that pharmacodynamic rather than pharmacokinetic studies are needed to deal with this question. There is apparently no danger in giving acute treatment at high dosage, because osteoblast activity will not be affected for the first month or two, as noted above.

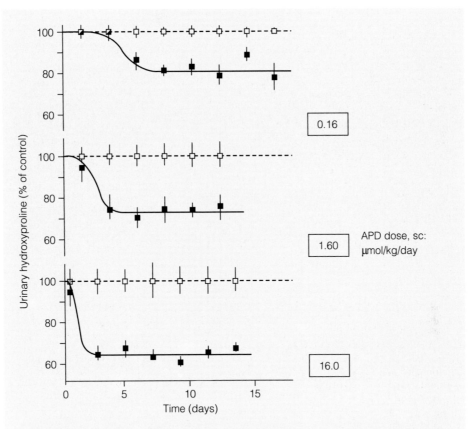

Fig. 7. Rate and degree of bone resorption suppression in groups of six rats, treated for 16 days with daily subcutaneous injections of pamidronate. Bone resorption is assessed as the urinary excretion of hydroxyproline, expressed as percentage of control values (mean ± s.e. mean). *Closed symbols* and *curve* are treated animals, *open symbols* and *interrupted curve* are controls (data after REITSMA et al, 1983).

Practical applications

Acute suppression of bone resorption is clearly indicated – in the light of the mechanisms by which bisphosphonates act – in patients with hypercalcaemia of malignancy, bone metastases, Paget's disease, and other causes of elevated bone resorption. As shown in Figures 7 and 9, most patients with Paget's disease can be brought into remission within a few months of starting bisphosphonate therapy. Many different treatment schedules have been used, but those studies in which 200 mg pamidronate has been given intravenously in divided doses over the first two to four weeks show the best results.

Bisphosphonates can however also be used in long-term modulation of bone remodelling – again in a range of indications, including osteoporosis, osteogenesis imperfecta, and steroid-induced osteoporosis. As supportive therapy

23

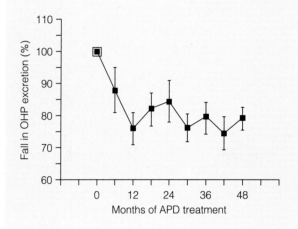

Fig. 8. Degree of bone resorption suppression in eight patients with osteoporosis, treated during four years with daily oral administration of 150 mg pamidronate. Bone resorption is assessed as the urinary excretion of hydroxyproline (OHP), expressed as percentage of pretreatment values (mean ± s.e. mean) (unpublished data after VALKEMA et al, 1989).

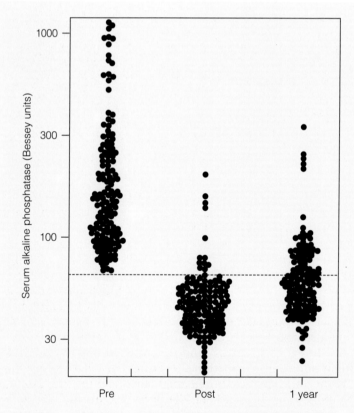

Fig. 9. Serum alkaline phosphatase activity in 142 patients with Paget's disease before treatment with pamidronate, at the end of treatment, and one year later (data after HARINCK et al, 1987c).

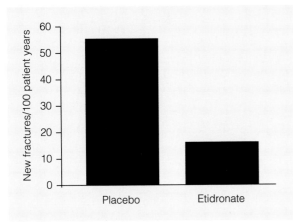

Fig. 10. Rate of new vertebral fractures in patients treated with etidronate, compared with placebo-treated controls. (Preliminary data from STORM et al, 1989a, with permission.)

Table II. Effect of pamidronate on bone metastases.

	Complication rate (per 100 patient years)		
	Total	Isolated	Combined
Treated with APD (*n* = 85)	52	43	9
Not treated with APD (*n* = 85)	94	59	35
	Patient rate (per 100 patient years)		
Treated with APD (*n* = 85)	34		
Not treated with APD (*n* = 85)	43		

of bone tumours, they can be given for secondary prevention or possibly even as adjuvant therapy, i.e. for primary prevention.

Preliminary results of recent studies (GENANT et al, 1989a, 1989b; STORM et al, 1989a, 1989b) provide reassuring evidence about the risk of fractures on long-term, low-dose bisphosphonate therapy. Patients on etidronate given (cyclically) 400 mg orally per day during two out of 15 weeks had a significantly reduced vertebral fracture rate compared with placebo-treated controls. Pamidronate seems likely to produce a similar response, since it has been shown to increase bone mass by 3% annually in patients with osteoporosis on oral treatment with 150 mg per day.

Finally, the preventive value of pamidronate in metastatic bone disease is shown in Table II, which portrays the complication rates attributable to bone metastases per 100 patient years in a group of 85 patients, compared with 85 controls not given pamidronate. The event rate is reduced by about 40% and the patient rate by over 20%. The larger reduction in event rate than in patient rate implies that complications, when occurring in the APD group, were less severe and less frequent per patient than in the control group. Neurometastatic disease was also reduced, though by less. Grading the lesions showed that those in the APD-treated group were generally less severe than among the controls. The full results (VAN HOLTEN-VERZANTVOORT, 1990; VAN HOLTEN-VERZANTVOORT et al, 1987) indicate a valuable preventive role for bisphosphonates in patients with malignant disease likely to metastasise to bone.

References

BARON, R., VIGNERY, A. and HOROWITZ, M. (1984) Lymphocytes, macrophages and the regulation of bone remodeling. In: *Bone and Mineral Research Annual 2*, W. A. Peck (Ed.), pp. 175–243. Elsevier, Amsterdam.

BIJVOET, O. L. M., FRIJLINK, W. B., JIE, K. et al (1980) APD in Paget's disease of bone. Role of the mononuclear phagocyte system? *Arthritis Rheum. 23*, 1193–1204.

BOONEKAMP, P. M., VAN DER WEE-PALS, L. J. A., VAN WIJK-VAN LENNEP, M. et al (1986) Two modes of action of bisphosphonates on osteoclastic resorption of mineralised matrix. *Bone Min. 1*, 27–40.

BOONEKAMP, P. M., LÖWIK, C. W. G. M., VAN DER WEE-PALS, L. J. A. (1987) Enhancement of the inhibitory action of APD on the transformation of osteoclast precursors into resorbing cells after dimethylation of the amino group. *Bone Min. 2*, 29–42.

CECCHINI, M. G., FELIX, R., FLEISCH, H. et al (1987) Effects of bisphosphonates on proliferation and viability of mouse bone-marrow derived macrophages. *J. Bone Min. Res. 2*, 135–142.

FLANAGAN, A. M. and CHAMBERS, T. J. (1989) Dichloromethylenebisphosphonate (C12MBP) inhibits resorption through injury to osteoclasts that resorb C12MBP-coated bone. *Bone Min. 6*, 33–43.

FLEISCH, H. (1983) Bisphosphonates: Mechanism of action and clinical application. In: *Bone and Mineral Research Annual 1*, W. A. Peck (Ed.), pp. 319–357. Elsevier, Amsterdam.

FLORA, L., HASSING, G. S., LLOYD, G. G. et al (1981) The long-term skeletal effects of EHDP in dogs. *Metab. Bone Dis. Rel. Res. 4*, 289–300.

FRANCIS, M. D. and MARTODAM, R. R. (1983) Chemical, biochemical and medicinal properties of the diphosphonates. In: *The Role of Phosphonates in Living Systems*, R. L. Hildebrand (Ed.), pp. 55–96. CRC Press Inc, Boca Raton, Florida.

FRIJLINK, W. B., TE VELDE, J., BIJVOET, O. L. M. et al (1979) Treatment of Paget's disease of bone with (3-amino-1-hydroxypropylidene)-1,1-bisphosphonate (APD). *Lancet i*, 799–803.

GENANT, H. K., HARRIS, S. T., STEIGER, P. et al (1989a) The effect of etidronate therapy in postmenopausal osteoporotic women: Preliminary results. In: *Osteoporosis 2*, C. Christiansen et al (Eds). pp. 177–181. Osteopress ApS, Copenhagen.

GENANT, H. K., HARRIS, S., DAVEYS, P. F. et al (1989b) The effect of cyclic etidronate therapy with or without phosphate in postmenopausal osteoporotic women: Three-year study results. In: *Cyclical Etidonate. A New Dimension in Therapy for Osteoporosis*, Grand Hotel, Paris, April 1989 (in press).

HARINCK, H. I. J., BIJVOET, O. L. M., BLANKSMA, H. J. et al (1987a) Efficacious management with aminobisphosphonate (APD) in Paget's disease of bone. *Clin. Orthop. 217*, 79–98.

HARINCK, H. I. J., BIJVOET, O. L. M., PLANTINGH, A. S. T. et al (1987b) The role of bone and kidney in tumor hypercalcemia and its treatment with bisphosphonate and sodium chloride. *Am. J. Med. 82*. 1133–1142.

HARINCK, H. I. J., PAPAPOULOS, S. E., BLANKSMA, H. J. et al (1987c) Paget's disease of bone: early and late responses to three different modes of treatment with aminohydroxypropylidene bisphosphonate (APD). *Br. Med. J. 295*, 1301–1305.

HORTON, M. A. (1988) Osteoclast specific antigens. *ISI Atlas of Science: Immunology*, 35–43.

HUGHES, D. E., MACDONALD, B. R., RUSSELL, R. G. et al (1989) Inhibition of osteoclast-like cell formation by bisphosphonates in long-term cultures of human bone marrow. *J. Clin. Invest. 83*, 1930–1935.

JAWORSKI, Z. G. F., DUCK, B. and SEKALY, G. (1981) Kinetics of osteoclasts and their nuclei in evolving secondary Haversian systems. *J. Anat. 133*, 397–405.

LERNER, U. H. and LARSSON, Å. (1987) Effects of four bisphosphonates on bone resorption, lysosomal enzyme release, protein synthesis and mitotic activities in mouse calvarial bones in vitro. *Bone 8*, 179–189.

LÖWIK, C. W. G. M., VAN DER PLUYM, G., VAN DER WEE-PALS, L. J. A. et al (1988) Migration and phenotypic transformation of osteoclast precursors into mature osteoclasts: the effects of a bisphosphonate. *J. Bone Min. Res. 2*, 185–192.

MORTON, A. R., CANTRILL, J. A., PILLAI, G. V. et al (1988) Sclerosis of lytic bone metastases after disodium aminohydroxypropylidene bisphosphonate (APD) in patients with breast carcinoma. *Br. Med. J. 297*, 772–773.

NIJWEIDE, P. J., BURGER, E. H. and FEYEN, J. H. M. (1986) The cells of bone: proliferation, differentiation and hormonal regulation. *Physiol. Rev. 66*, 855–886.

RAISZ, L. G. (1988) Local and systemic factors in the pathogenesis of osteoporosis. *N. Engl. J. Med. 318*, 818–828.

REITSMA, P. H., BIJVOET, O. L. M., VERLINDEN-OOMS, H. et al (1980) Kinetic studies of bone and mineral metabolism during treatment with (3-amino-1-hydroxypropylidene)-1,1-bisphosphonate (APD) and disodium dichloromethylene bisphosphonate (C12MDP) on rat macrophage mediated bone resorption in vitro. *J. Clin. Invest. 70*, 927–933.

REITSMA, P. H., BIJVOET, O. L. M., POTOKAR, M. et al (1983) Apposition and resorption of bone during oral treatment with (3-amino-1-hydroxypropylidene)-1,1-bisphosphonate (APD). *Calcif. Tissue Int. 35*, 357–361.

STORM, T. L., THAMSBORG, G., SØRENSEN, O. H. et al (1989a) The effects of etidronate therapy in postmenopausal osteoporotic women. Preliminary results. In: *Osteoporosis 2*, C. Christiansen et al (Eds), pp. 1172–1176. Osteopress ApS, Copenhagen.

STORM, T. L., THAMSBORG, G. and SØRENSEN, O. H. (1989b) The effect of etidonate cyclical therapy in postmenopausal osteoporosis. In: *Cyclical Etidronate. A New Dimension in Therapy for Osteoporosis.* Grand Hotel, Paris, April, 1989 (in press).

VALKEMA, R., VISMANS, F. J. F. E., PAPAPOULOS, S. E. et al (1989) Maintained improvement in calcium balance and bone mineral content in patients with osteoporosis treated with the bisphosphonate APD. *Bone Min. 5*, 183–192.

VAN HOLTEN-VERZANTVOORT, A. T., BIJVOET, O. L. M., CLETON, F. J. et al (1987) Reduced morbidity from skeletal metastases in breast cancer patients during long-term bisphosphonate (APD) treatment. *Lancet ii*, 983–985.

VAN HOLTEN-VERZANTVOORT, A. T. et al (1990) (in preparation).

Tumour-induced hypercalcaemia

Clinical efficacy of pamidronate (APD) in tumour-induced hypercalcaemia

P. Burckhardt (speaker), D. Thiébaud, P. Jaeger, L. Portmann and
A. F. Jacquet
Department of Internal Medicine, Centre Hospitalier Universitaire Vaudois,
Lausanne, Switzerland

Summary

Nine studies testing the efficacy of pamidronate (APD) in the treatment of hypercalcaemia of malignancy are presented. The studies investigate the optimum intravenous dosage and treatment schedules for APD, the effectiveness of oral therapy, the problems associated with second and subsequent courses of APD, and the use of APD and calcitonin together. APD is a safe and easy treatment for hypercalcaemia, suitable for about two-thirds of affected patients.

Introduction

The use of pamidronate (APD) in the treatment of Paget's disease showed it to be especially efficient in inhibiting bone resorption (Frijlink et al, 1979). Other studies (Yates et al, 1985; Atkins et al, 1987; Thiébaud et al, 1987) indicated that the effects of bisphosphonates were prolonged, even after very short periods of treatment. We therefore decided to test the efficacy of APD in tumour-induced hypercalcaemia, concentrating on dosage, route of administration and treatment schedules. The results of our studies are presented below.

Study 1

To evaluate the efficacy of intravenous APD in tumour-induced hypercalcaemia, 14 hypercalcaemic (average initial plasma calcium 3.38 mmol/l) patients were treated with APD 25 mg/day after hydration for 36–48 hours until the plasma calcium level was normal (less than 2.5 mmol/l) on two consecutive days (Portmann et al, 1983). No antitumour treatment was given during this period. The plasma calcium returned to normal in all patients, on average after three days (mean duration of treatment 5.6 days). Since the slope of the decrease was almost constant, duration of treatment depended essentially on the initial plasma calcium level.

Conclusion. APD normalises the plasma calcium in all hypercalcaemic patients, the time taken depending on the initial plasma calcium level.

Study 2

To determine if APD is equally effective when given orally, two groups of patients with tumour-induced hypercalcaemia were treated with either 30 mg APD per day intravenously (group A), or with 1200 mg APD per day orally (group B), for six days each (THIÉBAUD et al, 1986a). No antitumour treatment was given during this period. The average initial plasma calcium was 3.42 mmol/l in group A and 3.28 mmol/l in group B. Mean plasma calcium levels in both groups returned to normal within five days, though one patient with a very high initial plasma calcium (5.0 mmol/l) took eight days.

Conclusion. A total dose of 180 mg APD given intravenously over six days has the same effect on plasma calcium as a dose 40 times bigger given orally. Both treatments normalise the plasma calcium in all cases.

Study 3

Since all patients in the previous study became normocalcaemic on 180 mg APD intravenously it was possible that this dose was supra-optimal, and that a single infusion of 60 mg or less might be sufficient (THIÉBAUD et al, 1986b). To investigate this, 20 patients with tumour-induced hypercalcaemia were divided equally into two groups. One group received 30 mg APD intravenously, the other 60 mg, both given in 1 litre normal saline over 24 hours. No antitumour treatment was given during this period. Mean initial plasma calcium levels were 3.24 mmol/l and 3.22 mmol/l respectively.

In all patients treated with 60 mg APD, the plasma calcium returned to normal after 2–5 days, depending on the initial level. All patients receiving 30 mg APD responded, but in the three with the highest initial levels (less than 3.5 mmol/l), the plasma calcium did not return to normal. Two weeks after the 30 mg dose the plasma calcium began to rise slightly in most patients, but not after the 60 mg dose (Fig. 1). The same phenomenon was seen with urinary parameters. After the 30 mg dose both hydroxyproline excretion and to a lesser extent calcium excretion decreased sharply, but began to rise again after six days; this was not seen after the 60 mg dose.

Conclusion. When given as a single intravenous infusion, 30 mg APD are as effective in mild hypercalcaemia as 180 mg; severe cases need 60 mg. Inhibition of bone resorption, as evaluated by urinary hydroxyproline and calcium excretion, lasts longer after 60 mg than after 30 mg.

Study 4

Since the previous study showed 30 mg APD to be less effective than 60 mg in severe hypercalcaemia, we decided to use 45 and 90 mg APD as a single intravenous infusion over 24 hours, to see if a dose-response curve could be established (THIÉBAUD et al, 1988 a and b). Two further groups of patients with tumour-induced hypercalcaemia (ten patients per group) were treated with a single infusion of 45 or 90 mg APD and compared with the patients in the previous study.

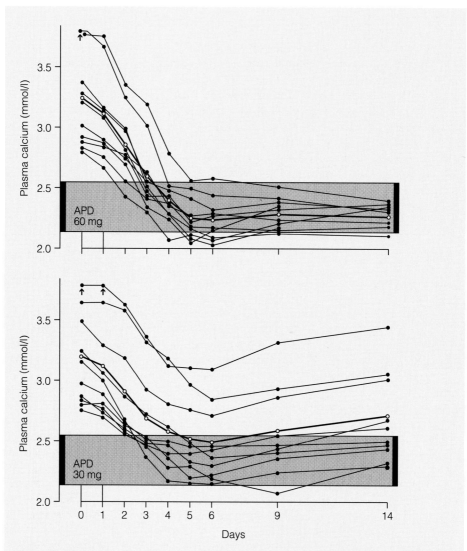

Fig. 1. Plasma calcium, corrected for proteins, in two groups of patients with tumour-induced hypercalcaemia, before and after a single dose of pamidronate (APD) 60 mg (upper panel) or 30 mg (lower panel). The open circles show the mean values, the shaded area the normal range of plasma calcium (2.15–2.55 mmol/l) (from THIÉBAUD et al, 1986b).

Plasma calcium returned to normal in all patients whose initial level was below 3.5 mmol/l; eight became transiently hypocalcaemic, either because of their initial plasma calcium (less than 3.0 mmol/l) or a relatively high dose of APD. Plasma calcium did not return completely to normal in eight of 24 patients with a high initial plasma calcium (more than 3.5 mmol/l) treated with 30 or 45 mg, but in only one of 14 patients given the higher doses.

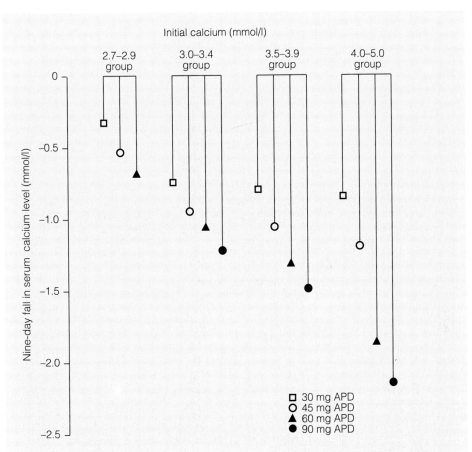

Fig. 2. Fall in plasma calcium over nine days following a single infusion of four different doses of APD in 40 patients with tumour-induced hypercalcaemia. Patients are grouped according to their initial plasma calcium level (modified from THIÉBAUD et al, 1988b).

When patients with similar initial plasma calcium levels were compared, the fall in serum calcium was dose dependent (Fig. 2), as were the falls in urinary excretion of calcium and hydroxyproline. The latter began to increase slightly nine days after the lower doses of APD, but were still declining two weeks after 90 mg APD. The follow-up study showed an identical survival rate in the four groups, of 30–50% after three months, but the recurrence rate of hypercalcaemia was strikingly different – only 30–40% after high doses of APD, compared with 60–80% after low doses.

Conclusion. Patients with severe hypercalcaemia need higher doses than those with mild hypercalcaemia (Fig. 3). Inhibition of bone resorption lasts longer after higher doses of APD than after low doses, even when administered as a single infusion.

Dose of APD

Initial plasma calcium (mmol/l)	30 mg	45 mg	60 mg	90 mg
4.0–5.0	×	× ×	× ●● ●●	●● ●●
3.5–3.9	× × ×	× × ●●	●● ● ●●	●● ●●
3.0–3.4	●● ●●	●● ●●	●● ● ◇	●● ◇ ◇
2.7–2.9	●● ● ◇	●● ● ◇	●● ◇ ◇ ◇	

Fig. 3. Summary of the changes in plasma calcium, as a function of the initial plasma calcium level, in 52 patients with tumour-induced hypercalcaemia treated with a single infusion of pamidronate (APD) at various doses. One symbol indicates one patient. Results of treatment: ● normal calcium; × slight hypercalcaemia; ◇ hypocalcaemia (from THIÉBAUD et al, 1988a).

Study 5

To see if there was an average minimum total dose of APD required to normalise plasma calcium across all tumour types and all degrees of hypercalcaemia, we reviewed the literature, picking out all studies where the dose and outcome of treatment were indicated (BURCKHARDT et al, 1989). In all, some 358 patients were identified; those given the same dose of APD were grouped together.

This study showed that a total dose of 90–100 mg APD achieved normocalcaemia in all patients, but that with lower doses the success rate was dose-dependent.

Conclusion. When the duration of intravenous treatment is progressively shortened, finally to a single 24-hour infusion, not all patients with severe hypercalcaemia achieve a normal plasma calcium with only 30 mg APD. Higher doses (60 mg and 90 mg) are more efficient, and also result in a more prolonged inhibition of bone resorption, as shown by decreased hydroxyproline excretion and the incidence of recurrent hypercalcaemia.

Study 6

To determine whether APD can be given repeatedly in recurrent hypercalcaemia without loss of efficacy, the results of a second course were compared with those of the first course in 12 patients with tumour-induced hypercalcaemia treated with the same dose of APD when their hypercalcaemia relapsed (THIÉBAUD et al, 1990a). The mean dose was 53 mg given as a single infusion, and the mean time between the two treatments was 35 days.

Mean initial plasma and urinary calcium levels were identical, but urinary hydroxyproline excretion was slightly higher when the hypercalcaemia relapsed. Response to APD was slightly less marked following the second course; although plasma calcium fell in every case, fewer patients reached a normal level. Urinary hydroxyproline decreased by a similar amount, but began to increase again slightly sooner. Renal handling of calcium was identical, and was not modified by the treatment.

Conclusion. APD can be used in recurrent hypercalcaemia, although its efficacy is slightly weaker. This is not due to an increase in the tubular reabsorption of calcium, but rather to decreased responsiveness and progression of the resorptive process in bone.

Study 7

Has the increased tubular reabsorption of calcium – an important pathophysiological mechanism of tumour-induced hypercalcaemia (MARTIN, 1988) – any relevance for the response to APD? To investigate this, the response to a single infusion of APD was compared in two groups of patients with significant differences in their tubular reabsorption of calcium: 20 patients with squamous cell carcinoma of the lung (eight with bone metastases), and 23 patients with breast cancer (all with metastases) (THIÉBAUD et al, 1990a). Mean initial plasma calcium levels were similar (3.40 and 3.37 mmol/l), while the mean tubular reabsorption of calcium (TmCa/GFR) was significantly different (2.58 ± 0.06 and 2.20 ± 0.05 mmol/l respectively). The average dose of APD was identical (57 and 56 mg).

The drop in plasma calcium levels in response to APD was the same in both groups. The TmCa/GFR values remained different, and were not modified by the treatment.

Conclusion. Increased tubular reabsorption of calcium does not diminish the response to APD, which is mainly conditioned by the inhibitory effect of bone resorption.

Study 8

Although inhibition of bone resorption by APD is quite sufficient to normalise the plasma calcium, even in the presence of increased tubular reabsorption of calcium, any treatment (such as calcitonin) which increases calciuria might contribute to the effects of APD (RALSTON et al, 1989). Is combined treatment with APD and calcitonin more effective because of this additional calciuric effect?

Seventeen hypercalcaemic patients with various tumours were treated with APD ± 53 mg, and 200 i.u. salmon calcitonin per day, given as suppositories over three days (provided by Sandoz Ltd, Basle, Switzerland) (THIÉBAUD et al, 1990b). Their biochemical responses were compared with a group of patients receiving only APD matched for initial plasma calcium, tumour type and dose of APD given, and selected from patients taking part in previous studies.

As expected, plasma calcium levels dropped significantly faster when calcitonin was given with APD. Urinary hydroxyproline excretion declined in both groups similarly, but urinary calcium excretion showed a sharper increase in patients treated with APD and calcitonin, and a fall in TmCa/GFR.

Conclusion. Although APD has a potent effect on hypercalcaemia by inhibiting bone resorption, the addition of calcitonin accelerates normalisation of plasma calcium by increasing urinary calcium excretion.

Study 9

As APD is a safe and effective treatment for tumour-induced hypercalcaemia, should it be used in every case?

Fifty consecutive hypercalcaemic patients with inoperable malignant disease were studied. In 14 cases, treatment of the hypercalcaemia was considered inappropriate because of endstage disease and imminent death. Treatment was arbitrarily considered as not indicated when the plasma calcium level was below 2.87 mmol/l (11.5 mg/100 ml), and was not undertaken for this reason in 20 patients. In four patients, severe renal insufficiency was considered a contraindication to treatment with bisphosphonates. Altogether, hypercalcaemia was treated in only 12 patients, 24% of the total.

Conclusion. In this study, only one quarter of patients with tumour-induced hypercalcaemia were treated. If hypercalcaemia of all degrees, including recurrent hypercalcaemia, is considered an indication for treatment, then 29 out of 44 patients (66%) would have been treated.

Conclusion

A single infusion of APD can normalise all tumour-induced hypercalcaemias, provided that the dose is adapted to the level of the hypercalcaemia. Response to a second dose of APD is slightly weaker. The immediate response does not depend on the tumour type, or on renal reabsorption of calcium, which is elevated in cases of humoral hypercalcaemia, especially when caused by secretion of PTH-related peptide. Since APD has no effect on urinary secretion of calcium, its calcium-lowering action can be enhanced when a calciuric drug such as calcitonin is administered concomitantly. These studies demonstrate the ease with which hypercalcaemia can be treated, and its suitability for about two-thirds of patients with tumour-induced hypercalcaemia.

References

ATKINS, R.M., YATES, A.J.P., GRAY, R.E.S. et al (1987) Aminohexane diphosphonate in the treatment of Paget's disease of bone. *J. Bone Min. Res. 2*, 273–279.

BURCKHARDT, P., THIÉBAUD, D., PEREY, L. et al (1989) Treatment of tumor-induced osteolysis by APD. In: *Bisphosphonates and Tumor Osteolysis. Recent Results in Cancer Research*, Vol. 116, K.W. Brunner et al (Eds), pp. 54–66. Springer, Berlin.

FRIJLINK, W.B., BIJVOET, O.L.M., TE VELDE, J. et al (1979) Treatment of Paget's disease with 3-amino-hydroxypropylidene-1-1-bisphosphonate (APD). *Lancet i*, 799–803.

MARTIN, T. J. (1988) Humoral hypercalcemia of malignancy. *Bone Min. 4*, 83–89.

PORTMANN, L., HÄFLIGER, J. M., BILL, G. et al (1983) Un traitement simple de l'hypercalcémie tumorale: l'amino-hydroxypropylidène bisphosphonate (APD) i.v. *Schweiz. Med. Wochenschr. 113*, 1960–1963.

RALSTON, S. H., BOYCE, B. F., COWAN, R. A. et al (1989) Contrasting mechanisms of hypercalcemia in patients with early and advanced humoral hypercalcemia of malignancy. *J. Bone Min. Res. 4*, 103–111.

THIÉBAUD, D., PORTMANN, L., JAEGER, P. et al (1986a) Oral versus intravenous AHPrBP in the treatment of hypercalcemia of malignancy. *Bone 7*, 247–253.

THIÉBAUD, D., JAEGER, P., JACQUET, A. F. et al (1986b) A single-day treatment of tumor-induced hypercalcemia by intravenous amino-hydroxypropylidene bisphosphonate. *J. Bone Min. Res. 1*, 555–562.

THIÉBAUD, D., JAEGER, P. and BURCKHARDT, P. (1987) Paget's disease of bone treated in five days with AHPrBP (APD) per os. *J. Bone Min. Res. 2*, 45–52.

THIÉBAUD, D., JAEGER, P., JACQUET, A. F. et al (1988a) Dose-response in the treatment of hypercalcemia of malignancy by a single infusion of the bisphosphonate AHPrBP. *J. Clin. Oncol. 6*, 762–768.

THIÉBAUD, D., JAEGER, P., JACQUET, A. F. et al (1988b) Traitement de l'hypercalcémie tumorale par un diphosphonate en perfusion unique. *Schweiz. Med. Wochenschr. 118*, 77–81.

THIÉBAUD, D., JAEGER, PH. and BURCKHARDT, P. (1990a) Response to retreatment of malignant hypercalcemia with the bisphosphonate AHPrBP (APD); respective role of kidney and bone. *J. Bone Min. Res.* (in press).

THIÉBAUD, D., JACQUET, A. F. and BURCKHARDT, P. (1990b) Fast and effective treatment of severe malignant hypercalcemia: combination of suppositories of calcitonin and single infusion of the bisphosphonate APD (AHPrBP). *Arch. Int. Med.* (in press).

YATES, A. J. P., GRAY, R. E. S., URWIN, G. H. et al (1985) Intravenous clodronate in the treatment and retreatment of Paget's disease of bone. *Lancet i*, 1474–1477.

Discussion

Dr R. E. COLEMAN (Edinburgh): When considering the duration of normocalcaemia after intravenous pamidronate it is very important to allow for the effect of changes in systemic treatment. Can you clarify whether changes in hormone or cytotoxic treatment have been allowed for, and that the normocalcaemia is entirely attributable to pamidronate?

BURCKHARDT: All the acute studies were completed before any antitumoural treatment was begun. This was in fact the major difficulty of using this protocol. The six-month and nine-month follow-up studies obviously did not permit us to sort out the effects of other treatments, though these usually remained unchanged during the period of observation. To be sure that the effects are exclusively attributable to APD is difficult in long-term studies.

The role of intravenous disodium pamidronate in the treatment of cancer-associated hypercalcaemia: comparison with conventional agents and other bisphosphonates

S. H. RALSTON

Rheumatic Diseases Unit, Northern General Hospital, Edinburgh, UK

Summary

Intravenous disodium pamidronate (APD) is a more effective treatment for cancer-associated hypercalcaemia than rehydration alone. Earlier studies have shown it to have a more sustained and more profound calcium-lowering action than either mithramycin or combined steroids and calcitonin in cancer-associated hypercalcaemia. As other bisphosphonates have also been shown to be effective in this condition, we compared response to pamidronate, etidronate and clodronate in 48 patients with hypercalcaemia of malignancy in excess of 2.80 mmol/l. Preliminary results suggest that pamidronate produces a more marked and better sustained fall in serum calcium than the other agents.

Introduction

In recent years intravenous disodium pamidronate (APD) has been shown to be an effective treatment for cancer-associated hypercalcaemia, significantly more effective than rehydration alone (SLEEBOOM et al, 1983). Although effective orally, pamidronate is poorly absorbed from the gut, and can cause gastrointestinal upset. Moreover, the frequent occurrence of nausea and vomiting in patients with cancer-associated hypercalcaemia and their almost invariable need for intravenous fluid therapy, makes parenteral administration more convenient.

Background studies

Following these observations, intravenous pamidronate (15 mg daily for a median of six days) was compared with mithramycin (25 µg/kg twice daily) and combined corticosteroids (prednisolone 40 mg daily) and calcitonin (100 IU t.i.d.) in the treatment of cancer-associated hypercalcaemia (RALSTON et al, 1985). Following 48 hours' rehydration with intravenous saline, 39 patients were randomly allocated to receive one of the three treatments. Corticosteroids and calcitonin had the most rapid onset of action – serum calcium being reduced by 0.3 mmol/l over the first 24 hours – but this was poorly sustained. In comparison, pamidronate had a slower onset of action, but a more sustained effect during the follow-up period. Nine days after treatment, serum calcium levels were significantly lower in the pamidronate group than in either of the

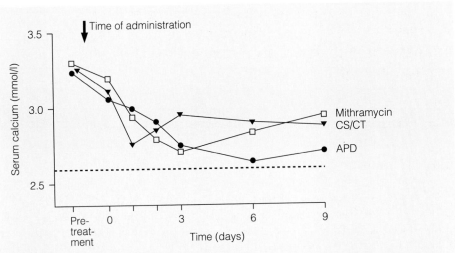

Fig. 1. Comparison of the effect of intravenous APD ($n = 13$), corticosteroid/calcitonin (CS/CT) ($n = 13$) and mithramycin ($n = 13$) on serum calcium in malignancy-associated hypercalcaemia. Values are medians. $P < 0.05$ between APD and other groups. Broken line = upper limit of normal range.

other groups (Fig. 1). Duration of effect (the time until further antihypercalcaemic therapy was needed) was also longer in the pamidronate group (average 20 days) than in either of the other groups (average 10–12 days).

After reports by Cantwell and Harris (1987). Thiébaud et al (1986) and Yates et al (1987) – showing encouraging results using single rather than multiple intravenous infusions of pamidronate in cancer-associated hypercalcaemia – we studied both the effects of single doses of pamidronate between 5 and 45 mg and the effect of varying the infusion time of a 45 mg dose over three, six and 24 hours (Ralston et al, 1988). With the exception of the 5 mg single dose, which was less effective (albeit not significantly so because of the small numbers), there was little to choose between single doses of 15–45 mg (Fig. 2). Infusion time did not affect response to the 45 mg dose. On this evidence we decided to use a single dose of 30 mg pamidronate as the routine initial treatment in further studies.

Other bisphosphonates

Bisphosphonates other than pamidronate have been shown to be effective in the treatment of cancer-associated hypercalcaemia. Hydroxyethylene bisphosphonate (etidronate) in doses of 7.5 mg/kg bodyweight/day for three days has been used successfully (Ryzen et al, 1985; Kanis et al, 1987), as has dichloromethylene bisphosphonate (clodronate) in doses of 300–600 mg daily for 1–10 days (Bonjour et al, 1988; Adami et al, 1987). These bisphosphonates are less potent in molar terms than pamidronate, and the doses used clinically are between 20 and 50 times higher to compensate for this. Does pamidronate's greater potency offer any advantage in terms of clinical efficacy?

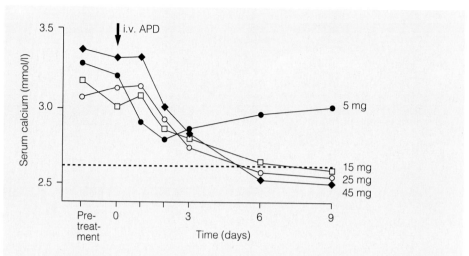

Fig. 2. Effect of different doses and response to single doses of intravenous APD in cancer-associated hypercalcaemia. There was little evidence of a dose-response relationship above 15 mg. Broken line = upper limit of normal range.

Patients and methods

To answer this question, we have recently compared the effects of intravenous pamidronate, clodronate and etidronate in 48 patients with cancer-associated hypercalcaemia in excess of 2.80 mmol/l. As in previous studies, patients were rehydrated for 48 hours prior to receiving a bisphosphonate – either pamidronate 30 mg over four hours, clodronate 600 mg over six hours, or etidronate 7.5 mg/kg/bodyweight/day for three days. These doses were chosen because they were in the middle of the range for the bisphosphonate in question, and previous experience had suggested that the dose was clinically effective. The study protocol is shown in Figure 3, and the spread of malignant conditions between the three treatment groups in Table I.

Results

Preliminary analysis of results indicates that all three bisphosphonates are effective in lowering serum calcium levels from those achieved by rehydration alone, with a maximum decline approximately six days after treatment in each case (Fig. 4). Full analysis is as yet incomplete, but the preliminary findings suggest that the calcium-lowering response is most marked and better sustained with pamidronate. Duration of effect is also significantly longer with pamidronate (median 29 days), compared to 13.5 days with clodronate ($P<0.05$) and 11 days with etidronate ($P<0.05$). Analysis of the mechanisms of action shows that all three agents inhibit bone resorption, but that this effect is most marked in pamidronate, so explaining its more potent calcium-lowering effects.

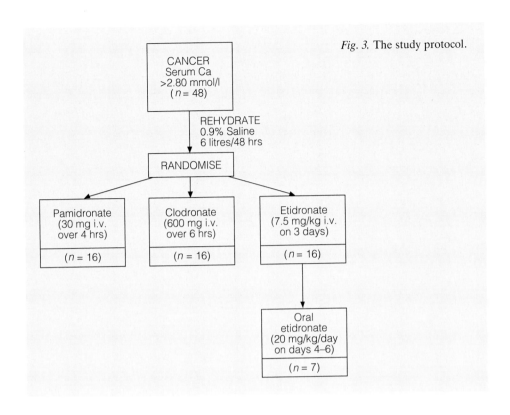

Fig. 3. The study protocol.

Discussion

Pamidronate is an effective calcium-lowering agent in most patients with cancer-associated hypercalcaemia. A relatively modest dose of 30 mg can achieve normocalcaemia in approximately 90% of patients during their first episode of hypercalcaemia. It is important to emphasise the marked between-centre variation in the rate of response to pamidronate, probably related to local differences in tumour type, the mechanism of hypercalcaemia in individual patients, and the degree of tumour advancement. For example, in a previous study, we achieved normocalcaemia in just over 50% of patients given an average dose of 90 mg pamidronate using the 15 mg daily Bijvoet regimen (SLEEBOOM et al, 1983), whereas HARINCK et al (1987) reported 90% normocalcaemia using an identical regimen. It has recently been suggested (GURNEY et al, 1989; RALSTON et al, 1987) that cancer patients with hypercalcaemia mediated by PTH-related peptides may respond less well to bisphosphonates and other antihypercalcaemic drugs than those with local osteolytic hypercalcaemia, and that this is likely to be a source of discrepancy when comparing success rates between different centres. In view of this, we suggest that the optimal dose of pamidronate may need to be determined on the basis of local experience and in the light of factors such as tumour type and stage.

41

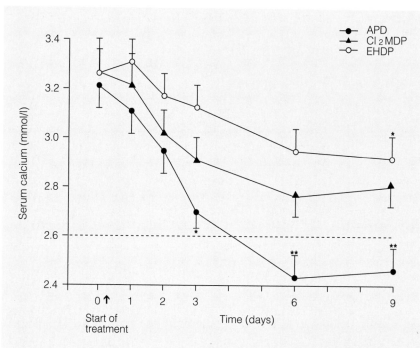

Fig. 4. Reduction in serum calcium levels in patients treated with pamidronate (APD), clodronate (Cl₂MDP) or etidronate (EHDP) following rehydration for 48 hours. Broken line = upper limit of normal range. *P<0.01 between APD and clodronate, **P<0.001 between APD and etidronate.

Table I. The distribution of malignant conditions between the three treatment groups.

	Pamidronate	Clodronate	Etidronate
Lung	6	6	7
Breast	4	3	3
Myeloma	2	1	1
Other	4	6	5
Total	16	16	16

Conclusion

Although some patients respond incompletely even to high doses of pamidronate, due to increased renal tubular reabsorption of calcium, in general the response to pamidronate is better than that achieved by other antihypercalcaemic agents, and is often accompanied by clinical improvement. Intravenous pamidronate seems the current treatment of choice for cancer-associated hypercalcaemia.

References

ADAMI, S., BOLZICCO, G. P., RIZZO, A. et al (1987) The use of dichloromethylene bisphosphonate and aminobutane bisphosphonate in hypercalcemia of malignancy. *Bone Min. 2,* 395–404.

BONJOUR, J. P., PHILIPPE, J., GUELPA, G. et al (1988) Bone and renal components in hypercalcemia of malignancy and responses to a single infusion of clodronate. *Bone 9,* 123–230.

CANTWELL, B. M. J. and HARRIS, A. L. (1987) Effect of single high dose infusions of aminohydroxypropylidene diphosphonate on hypercalcaemia caused by cancer. *Br. Med. J. 294,* 467–469.

GURNEY, H., KEFFORD, R. and STUART-HARRIS, R. (1989) Renal phosphate threshold and response to pamidronate in humoral hypercalcaemia of malignancy. *Lancet ii,* 241–243.

HARINCK, H. I., BIJVOET, O. L., PLANTINGH, A. S. et al (1987) Role of bone and kidney in tumor-induced hypercalcemia and its treatment with bisphosphonate and sodium chloride. *Am. J. Med. 82,* 1133–1142.

KANIS, J. A., URWIN, G. H., GRAY, R. E. et al (1987) Effects of intravenous etidronate disodium on skeletal and calcium metabolism. *Am. J. Med. 82* (Suppl. 2A), 55–70.

RALSTON, S. H., GARDNER, M. D., DRYBURGH, F. J. et al (1985) Comparison of aminohydroxypropylidene diphosphonate, mithramycin and corticosteroids/calcitonin in treatment of cancer-associated hypercalcaemia. *Lancet ii,* 907–910.

RALSTON, S. H., GARDNER, M. D., JENKINS, A. S. et al (1987) Malignancy-associated hypercalcemia: relationship between mechanisms of hypercalcemia and response to antihypercalcemic therapy. *Bone Min. 2,* 227–242.

RALSTON, S. H., ALZAID, A. A., GALLACHER, S. J. et al (1988) Clinical experience with amino-hydroxypropylidene bisphosphonate (APD) in the management of cancer-associated hypercalcaemia. *Q. J. Med. 69* (258), 825–834.

RYZEN, E., MARTODAM, R. R., TROXELL, M. et al (1985) Intravenous etidronate in the management of malignant hypercalcemia. *Arch. Int. Med. 145,* 449–452.

SLEEBOOM, H. P., BIJVOET, O. L. M., VAN OOSTEROM, A. T. et al (1983) Comparison of intravenous (3-amino-1-hydroxypropylidene)-1,1-bisphosphonate and volume repletion in tumour-induced hypercalcaemia. *Lancet ii,* 239–243.

THIÉBAUD, D., JAEGER, P. H. and BURCKHARDT, P. (1986) A single-day treatment of tumor-induced hypercalcemia by intravenous aminohydroxypropylidene bisphosphonate. *J. Bone Min. Res. 1,* 555–562.

YATES, A. J. P., MURRAY, R. M., JERUMS, G. J. et al (1987) A comparison of single and multiple intravenous infusion of 3-amino-1-hydroxypropylidene-1,1-bisphosphonate (APD) in the treatment of hypercalcaemia of malignancy. *Aust. N. Z. J. Med. 17,* 387–391.

Condensed paper

Pamidronate (APD) treatment of hypercalcaemia associated with malignancy – preliminary report of a multicentre double-blind trial

S. R. Nussbaum[1] (speaker), L. Mallette[2], R. Gagel[2], R. Chapman[3], G. Henderson[4] and C. Vandepol[5]

[1]Massachusetts General Hospital and Harvard Medical School, Boston, Massachusetts, [2]Baylor College of Medicine and Veterans Administration Medical Center, [3]Henry Ford Hospital, [4]Dana Farber Cancer Institute, and [5]Ciba-Geigy Corporation, Summit, New Jersey, USA

Malignancy is the most frequent underlying cause of hypercalcaemia among hospital inpatients. There are two main pathophysiological mechanisms: *osteolytic* due to metastases, and *humoral,* typically mediated by secretion of parathyroid hormone-related protein. The former mechanism is most often observed in breast carcinoma, the latter in squamous cancers. Both types share a common mechanism of calcium release – by osteoclastic resorption of bone.

Since the bisphosphonate compound pamidronate (APD) has been shown to inhibit osteoclast resorption of bone, there is a clear rationale for using it to treat hypercalcaemia, and several European studies have demonstrated the efficacy of a single intravenous infusion. To study the efficacy of different doses given in this way, we set up a four-centre randomised double-blind trial in which 30, 60 or 90 mg of APD was administered intravenously over 24 hours. Study subjects were carefully monitored in hospital for one week, then weekly for up to 60 days or until hypercalcaemia recurred.

Patients enrolled in this study had a histologically-confirmed malignancy with corrected serum calcium of at least 3.0 mmol/l (12.0 mg/100 ml), following 48 hours of saline hydration at 3.6 litres/24 hours. Exclusion criteria were significant renal impairment, other hypercalcaemic therapy during the week before entry into the study (although several patients had become resistant to alternative hypocalcaemic therapies, including plicamycin), and newly-initiated cancer chemotherapy. Efficacy was assessed by determining the duration of normocalcaemia, representing a complete response, and the time to relapse of hypercalcaemia (i.e. serum calcium above 2.9 mmol/l (11.5 mg/100 ml).

The majority of the 52 patients enrolled had skeletal metastases, though 16 had humoral hypercalcaemia without bone metastases. The most frequent tumours were lung cancer (in 26% of patients), breast cancer (18%), renal cancer (14%), head and neck cancer (8%) and haematological malignancies (10%).

Patients received 30, 60 or 90 mg APD as a 24-hour single infusion. In the 30 mg treatment group, the mean corrected serum calcium declined from 3.5 ($\pm$0.4) to 2.9 ($\pm$0.6) mmol/l, in the 60 mg group from 3.4 ($\pm$0.3) to 2.6 ($\pm$0.4) mmol/l and in the 90 mg group from 3.3 ($\pm$0.2) to 2.4 ($\pm$0.2) mmol/l (Fig. 1).

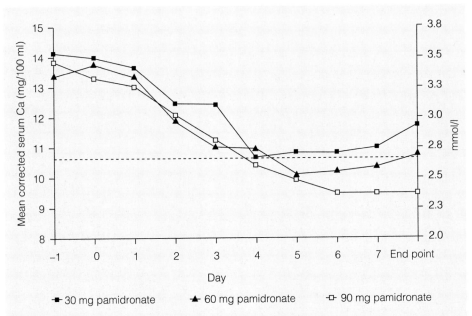

Fig. 1. Mean corrected serum calcium levels following a single infusion of APD (*n* = 52): comparison of 30, 60 and 90 mg doses.

The serum calcium was normalised in only 40% of patients who received 30 mg, in 61% of patients who received 60 mg, and in 100% of patients who received 90 mg of APD, though each treatment group initially had a similar high mean level of hypercalcaemia. The falls in serum calcium in each group were similar for patients with and without metastases and for different types of cancer. Complete response, often associated with marked clinical improvement, varied with the dose but lasted for as long as 2–3 months in patients with prolonged survival or following a second 60 mg infusion of pamidronate. Among the patients in each treatment group, the median duration of complete response was four, five and six days respectively for the 30, 60 and 90 mg doses. Side effects included transient asymptomatic hypocalcaemia, hypophosphataemia, and low-grade fever in some patients. There were no consistent haematological changes. Mean parathyroid-hormone levels were very low or undetectable before APD treatment and increased as normocalcaemia was achieved.

In conclusion, APD given as single 24-hour intravenous infusions of 30–90 mg appears to be both safe and effective in the treatment of hypercalcaemia of malignancy.

Discussion

Dr N. ROWELL (London): Are the hypophosphataemia and hypomagnesaemia sometimes attributed to bisphosphonate therapy of clinical relevance? Is it necessary to correct them?

45

NUSSBAUM: Correction is not generally necessary, unless phosphate levels fall below 1.5 mg/100 ml or magnesium levels below 0.8 mmol/l. Many patients with malignant disease have profound weakness and fatigue, which might be related, in part, to hypophosphataemia, but I do not think that it is often the significant factor. Hypophosphataemia may be exacerbated by bone remineralisation in areas of active resorption or by increased parathyroid hormone secretion with its phosphaturic action.

Professor O.L.M. BIJVOET (Leiden): Serum magnesium generally increases during bisphosphonate treatment, probably due to increased renal tubular absorption of magnesium – but some patients will have been magnesium-depleted by previous diuretic therapy. Hypomagnesaemia does not become more frequent at higher doses of APD, indicating that it is not APD related.

Condensed paper

Pamidronate (APD) and etidronate disodium (EHDP) in hypercalcaemia of malignancy – preliminary report of a comparative multicentre trial

P. Ritch[1] (speaker), R. Gucalp, P. Wiernik, P. Sarma, A. Keller,
S. Richman, K. Tauer, J. Neidhart, L. Mallette, R. Siegel and
C. Vandepol
[1]Hematology and Oncology Section, Medical College of Wisconsin,
Milwaukee, USA

A comparative trial of pamidronate (APD) and etidronate (EHDP) has been performed to determine their efficacy and tolerability in the treatment of hypercalcaemia of malignancy. About 10–20% of cancer patients develop hypercalcaemia during the course of their disease, mainly as a result of increased bone resorption. The bisphosphonates APD and EHDP are both potent inhibitors of bone resorption used successfully in the treatment of cancer-related hypercalcaemia. In the United States, etidronate is the only drug of this class at present available for routine clinical use. Because many excellent European studies have demonstrated high efficacy for pamidronate, we decided to set up a large-scale multicentre trial with two objectives:

– To compare the effect of intravenous APD and EHDP in lowering corrected serum calcium levels in cancer patients who had persistent hypercalcaemia after adequate hydration, and
– To evaluate the tolerability and safety of each drug.

The multicentre trial was conducted at nine institutions, using a randomised, parallel, double-blind, double-dummy design. A single 24-hour intravenous infusion containing APD 60 mg was compared to three consecutive daily infusions of EHDP containing the standard recommended dose of 7.5 mg/kg bodyweight/day (Table I).

Following initial screening and hydration with a minimum of three litres of normal saline over 24 hours, 65 patients with various types of malignancy and a corrected serum calcium of at least 3 mmol/l (12 mg/100 ml) after hydration were entered into the study and randomised to ADP or EHDP. On the first day of treatment, all patients received infusions containing one or other of the active drugs. On each of the subsequent two days, the APD patients received placebo infusions, to maintain the blindness of the study, whereas the EHDP patients received two further infusions containing the active drug. All patients were then monitored by means of follow-up examinations and laboratory studies, as indicated in Table I.

In addition to serum calcium of at least 3 mmol/l after adequate hydration, entry criteria included serum creatinine below 2.5 mg/100 ml and an estimated life-expectancy of at least one month, to permit follow-up evaluation. Patients who had recently received any other antihypercalcaemic therapy or newly-

Table I. Design of comparative trial.

Pre-study	Visit 1		Visits 2 and 3	Inpatient/outpatient follow-up
Hydration and screening	Intravenous infusion containing either:			
	APD 60 mg or EHDP 7.5 mg/kg		Placebo or EHDP 7.5 mg/kg	Weekly/monthly evaluation
Day: –1	0		1 and 2	3–7, 14, 21, 30

initiated cancer therapy were excluded from the study. Efficacy parameters included the serum calcium level, both measured and corrected, the duration of complete response to therapy, time to relapse, and major symptoms of hypercalcaemia.

Of the 65 patients who entered the study, 30 were randomly assigned to APD and 35 to EHDP; all were suitable for evaluation of efficacy and tolerability. The two groups were well balanced with respect to sex, age, presence or absence of bone metastases, and pretreatment serum calcium levels (measured and albumin-corrected). The two groups were also similar for tumour types, the most frequent being lung, breast, kidney, haematological, and head and neck malignancies.

The response was considered to be complete if the corrected serum calcium was in the normal range after bisphosphonate treatment. The complete response rates based on serum calcium determinations were 90% for patients in the APD group and 66% for those in the EHDP group, at the chosen dosage; after correction of serum calcium levels, complete response rates were 70% in the APD compared with 41% in the EHDP group ($P < 0.001$). After one week, 58% of the APD patients and 27% of the EHDP patients continued to have a complete response. Patients in the APD-treated group showed statistically greater reductions in mean serum calcium (measured and corrected) than those in the EHDP group.

The median duration of complete response (i.e. serum calcium below upper limit of normal range) was seven days in the APD and five days in the EHDP group. The median time to relapse of hypercalcaemia was 9.5 days in the APD and four days in the EHDP group.

The overall incidence of side effects was similar for the two treatment groups (30.0% for APD and 28.6% for EHDP), though fever was more frequent among APD (16.7%) than among EHDP patients (8.6%). One EHDP patient experienced new onset of seizures after treatment and one APD patient had hypocalcaemia reported as an adverse event.

In conclusion, APD is a safe and effective therapy for hypercalcaemia of malignancy. These preliminary findings suggest that it is statistically superior to EHDP in normalising serum calcium levels.

48

Discussion

Dr S. H. RALSTON (Edinburgh): Different centres using the same dose of APD get quite different responses. Were you able to analyse why some patients responded less well? Could this be due to tumour type, to failure to inhibit bone resorption, or to renal tubular reabsorption?

RITCH: These are preliminary results, and I have not yet seen a breakdown according to tumour type. With regard to response rates varying, there must be a considerable heterogeneity of patients, not just in terms of serum calcium but also in general condition and in standards of follow-up.

Dr J. P. ARMAND (Villejuif): Do you think it better to stratify tumour types in research, or to mix various types of disease together?

RITCH: Stratification is preferable, but studies should at least differentiate between hypercalcaemic conditions associated with a humoral mechanism and those where there is direct bone destruction.

Professor O. L. M. BIJVOET (Leiden): A so-called 'treatment failure' really means failure of the dosage schedule used – i.e. the total dose given may not be sufficient in relation to the initial severity of hypercalcaemia. In my experience, if normocalcaemia has not been achieved within five days, treatment should be continued for a few more days – until it is achieved.

RITCH: I agree. Clinically, it is essential to individualise therapy rather than use a standard schedule.

Bone metastases

Pamidronate (APD) treatment of bone metastases from breast cancer

R. E. COLEMAN

Imperial Cancer Research Fund, Medical Oncology Unit, Western General Hospital, Edinburgh, UK

Summary

The bisphosphonate pamidronate (APD) is a potent inhibitor of osteolysis, and the most effective agent available for treating hypercalcaemia of malignancy. The possibility that regular administration of pamidronate may result in long-term inhibition of osteoclast-induced bone resorption has been investigated.

Parenteral APD was given fortnightly to 28 patients with progressive bone metastases from breast cancer. No other systemic therapy was prescribed. APD prevented further bone destruction in 15 patients; four of these achieved a UICC partial response, while the remaining 11 showed no change on serial radiographs. The median duration of response (both groups) was six months (range 3–21). Symptomatic response was seen in nine patients.

A phase I study of a new, oral, effervescent formulation of APD suggested this might be more convenient than parenteral administration. Bone resorption was inhibited at doses below the threshold for gastrointestinal toxicity. Urinary calcium excretion fell to normal within two weeks in 14 out of 15 patients. Studies into the long-term tolerability of oral APD, and the use of APD as an adjunct to systemic treatment, are now indicated.

Introduction

The bisphosphonates are pyrophosphate analogues resistant to endogenous phosphatases. They contain a P–C–P structure which binds tightly to calcified bone matrix; some are potent inhibitors of osteoclast-induced bone resorption. Previous studies have shown that the bisphosphonates are effective in controlling Paget's disease, both disuse- and steroid-induced osteoporosis, and the hypercalcaemia of malignancy – conditions which are all characterised by increased rates of bone resorption. It is this inhibition of osteoclast-induced bone resorption which is of particular clinical relevance in the management of bone metastases in advanced breast cancer.

How bisphosphonates work is unclear; possible mechanisms include direct biochemical effects on the osteoclast, prevention of osteoclast attachment to the bone matrix or, in the case of pamidronate (APD), inhibition of osteoclast differentiation and recruitment (FLEISCH, 1988). Studies in murine tumours have shown that the bisphosphonates have neither a direct anticancer activity nor an effect on the efficacy of conventional anticancer drugs (GARATTINI et al,

1987). Similarly, immune function is not affected. The influence of APD on bone resorption, tumour growth in bone, metastasis formation and direct malignant invasion of bone is probably wholly attributable to its effects on osteoclast activity.

In addition to inhibiting bone resorption, bisphosphonates have the ability, in varying degrees, to block bone mineralisation. This has important clinical consequences. Etidronate (EHDP) inhibits mineralisation to the extent that osteomalacia and pathological fractures may occur. Clodronate (Cl_2MDP) has considerably less effect on mineralisation, but relatively high doses are required to inhibit osteolysis. Pamidronate (APD) is the most potent of the three, and inhibits bone resorption at low doses with minimal effects on mineralisation. Pamidronate also affects the mononuclear-phagocyte system – an action manifested by the fever and lymphopenia seen during the first week of administration (ADAMI et al, 1987) – and possibly inhibits the production of mature functional osteoclasts.

Our understanding of the pathogenesis of skeletal metastases is incomplete, but activation of osteoclasts is clearly relevant, providing a rationale for the use of inhibitors of bone resorption. Tumours secrete a variety of paracrine factors which stimulate bone cell activity, but in advanced breast cancer osteoclast activity usually predominates, and lytic bone metastases develop. The normal coupling between osteoclast and osteoblast results in some new bone formation, but despite this there is a net loss of calcium from the skeleton (Fig. 1).

Experimental evidence suggests that agents capable of reducing bone resorption might be of value in three ways:

– by inhibiting local osteolysis by the tumour, minimising structural damage and reducing the incidence of pain, pathological fracture and hypercalcaemia
– by protecting the bone from systemic mediators of resorption (humoral factors), and
– by decreasing the incidence of new metastatic lesions.

The results of two studies in patients with advanced breast cancer will be discussed. The first (COLEMAN et al, 1988) was a phase II study of parenteral APD given fortnightly for bone metastases, the second (COLEMAN et al, 1990) a phase I study of a new, oral, effervescent formulation of APD. No other systemic anticancer treatment was prescribed, allowing detailed assessment of objective, symptomatic and biochemical responses to APD.

The parenteral APD study

The optimum schedule and route of administration of pamidronate have not yet been defined and the dose-response relationship of single doses above 30 mg is disputed (BODY et al, 1987; THIÉBAUD et al, 1988). In our experience, a single intravenous dose of 15–30 mg pamidronate will control hypercalcaemia in 90% of patients for about two weeks (COLEMAN and RUBENS, 1987; COLEMAN and RUBENS, 1990); based on this data, an infusion of 30 mg pamidronate every two or three weeks seemed a suitable schedule for long-term outpatient use.

53

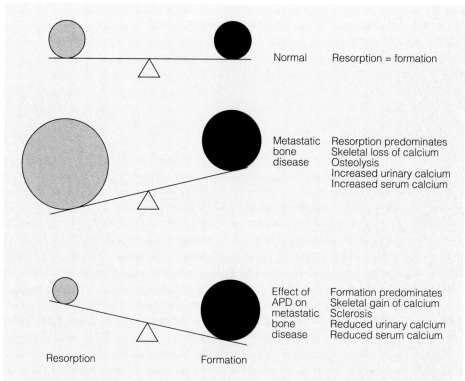

Normal — Resorption = formation

Metastatic bone disease — Resorption predominates Skeletal loss of calcium Osteolysis Increased urinary calcium Increased serum calcium

Effect of APD on metastatic bone disease — Formation predominates Skeletal gain of calcium Sclerosis Reduced urinary calcium Reduced serum calcium

Resorption   Formation

Fig. 1. The balance between bone resorption and formation. In health *(top)*, the normal coupling mechanisms ensure that bone turnover is balanced, but in metastatic bone disease *(middle)* the balance is disturbed, with resorption usually predominating. Treatment with APD selectively inhibits bone resorption, tipping the balance back in favour of bone formation *(bottom)* and promoting an increase in bone mass.

Twenty-eight patients received pamidronate as sole systemic therapy for breast cancer; all had radiological evidence of progressive lytic, or mixed lytic and sclerotic, bone metastases widely disseminated throughout the axial skeleton, and all had received previous systemic treatment. Objective response was assessed by UICC criteria, subjective response by a pain questionnaire, and biochemical response by serial measurements of serum calcium, osteocalcin (bone Gla-protein; Gla = gamma-carboxyglutamic acid), and urinary calcium excretion.

Pamidronate was given as an intravenous infusion in 500 ml normal (0.9%) saline over two hours every 14 days, and continued until progression of disease. The median number of APD treatments was eight (range 2–35). Painful sites of disease were treated with radiotherapy and analgesics were given as necessary.

Radiological evidence of bone healing was seen in four out of 24 evaluable patients (17%), in whom sclerosis of lytic lesions occurred with no evidence of new lesions. The sites undergoing sclerosis were outside the fields of previous radiotherapy. The median duration of response was ten months (range 9–21).

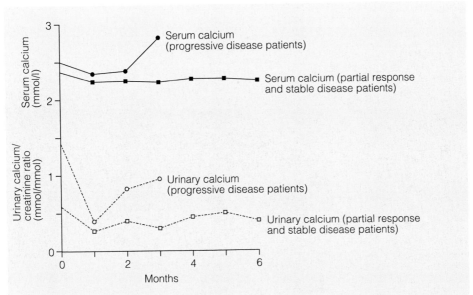

Fig. 2. Serial monthly values of serum calcium and the urinary calcium/creatinine ratio. Data shown separately for patients with responding or stable disease ($n = 15$) and those with progressive disease ($n = 9$).

Stabilisation of previously progressive bone disease for a minimum of three months (median five months, range 3–7 months) occurred in 11 patients (46%), including six in whom extraskeletal progression necessitated a change in treatment prior to any evidence of deteriorating skeletal disease. The median time to progressive bone disease was 16 weeks (range 5–90 weeks), although eight patients progressed within three months. The median duration of survival was eight months (range 1–36 months).

Nine patients showed a sustained symptomatic improvement in symptom score lasting more than six weeks; in five this was sufficiently marked to allow a major increase in mobility. All these patients remained pain free for more than a year, and four were able to stop opiate analgesics. Morbidity from bone metastases still occurred, and included pathological long-bone fracture (one patient), spinal cord compression (four patients), bone marrow infiltration (three patients), and hypercalcaemia (two patients).

Serial biochemical measurements indicated selective inhibition of osteolysis, with significant falls in serum calcium and urinary calcium levels (Fig. 2). The baseline values of both these parameters were highest in those patients who subsequently progressed on treatment, and although APD reduced urinary calcium excretion in 20 out of 24 patients irrespective of eventual outcome, the reduction was only sustained in those who responded to treatment or achieved stable disease. Despite inhibition of bone resorption there was no suggestion of inhibited osteoblast activity; indeed, serial osteocalcin levels increased in responding and stable patients, suggesting an increase in the rate of bone mineralisation (Fig. 3).

55

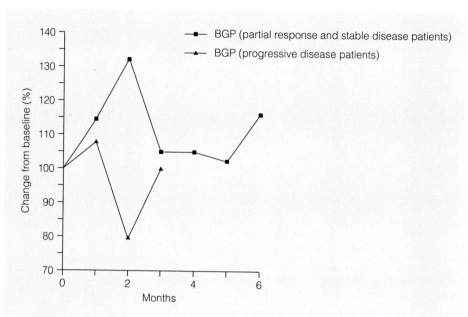

Fig. 3. Serial monthly values of osteocalcin (BGP). Data shown separately for patients with responding or stable disease ($n = 15$) and for those with progressive disease ($n = 9$).

APD was well tolerated and without serious toxicity. Possible drug-related side effects included elevation of liver transaminases in seven patients, mild pyrexia, lymphopenia and hyperphosphataemia in two patients each, and an unexplained grand mal convulsion with reversible leucoencephalopathy in one patient.

The oral APD study

In the past the use of oral pamidronate has been limited by gastrointestinal intolerance due to its corrosive properties, poor absorption from the bowel and binding to dietary calcium. New oral formulations have recently been produced, including enteric-coated and effervescent tablets. The latter form a true solution in water, thus avoiding the high local concentration of APD in the upper gastrointestinal tract which occurs with ordinary tablets or a suspension. Nineteen patients with progressive bone metastases from breast cancer were studied; 15 had evidence of increased osteolysis, with a urinary calcium excretion in excess of 0.4 mmol/mmol creatinine. The first four patients received 150 mg APD daily for four weeks; subsequent cohorts of four patients received APD 300 mg, 450 mg or 600 mg daily. In two of the patients with normal urinary calcium excretion the dose was increased weekly to a maximum of 600 mg daily. APD was taken dissolved in water at least one hour before food

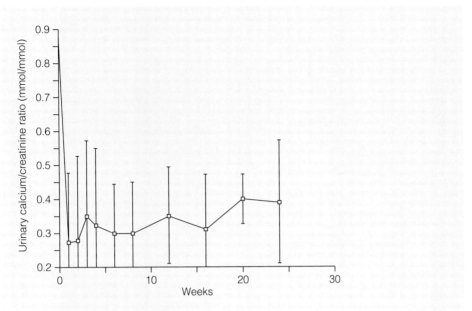

Fig. 4. Urinary calcium/creatinine ratios following oral APD in doses between 150 and 600 mg daily (see text). All patients ($n = 15$) with raised baseline values are included. Mean values and standard error of the mean are shown.

or a milky drink. Patients were assessed weekly for the first month, both to record toxicity and to monitor biochemical levels. Treatment was continued beyond the four-week test period in patients who tolerated the treatment and reported symptomatic improvement. The median duration of treatment was ten weeks (range 3–29 weeks).

Within two weeks, 14 out of 15 patients showed a fall in urinary calcium excretion to normal, indicating adequate absorption of APD and inhibition of bone resorption at all dosages (Fig. 4). No significant difference in efficacy between the four doses was seen (Fig. 5). Serum calcium fell significantly but always remained within the normal range (Fig. 6). Nine out of 17 patients reported pain relief and were able to reduce their analgesics. Radiological follow-up was limited to the six patients who continued APD for more than four months. No change in the lytic component of their disease was seen, but one patient developed spinal cord compression due to epidural extension of tumour.

Oral APD was well tolerated at doses of 150 and 300 mg daily, but higher doses caused unacceptable nausea, vomiting and indigestion; three out of six patients on 450 mg daily and five out of six on 600 mg daily were unable to continue treatment. Gastrointestinal toxicity in these patients occurred within the first few weeks of treatment and resolved on stopping APD. No other toxicity was seen.

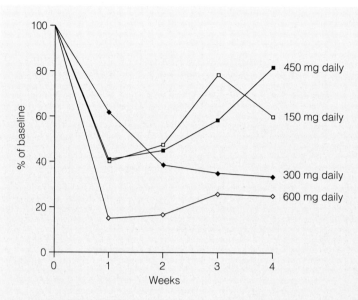

Fig. 5. The effect of different doses of APD on the urinary calcium/creatinine ratio. Data points represent the mean values of four patients at each dosage level.

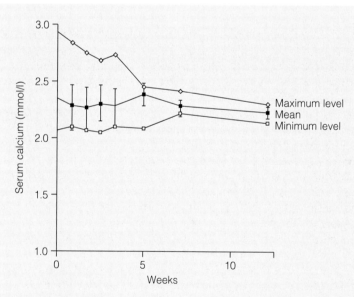

Fig. 6. Serum calcium levels following oral APD in doses between 150 and 600 mg daily ($n = 19$). Mean and standard error of the mean, and maximum and minimum values are shown.

The success of bisphosphonates in the management of hypercalcaemia of malignancy (BODY et al, 1987; SLEEBOOM et al, 1983) has encouraged study of their use in the long-term inhibition of bone resorption and for palliation of metastatic bone disease. Preliminary results suggest control of bone pain and a fall in urinary calcium and hydroxyproline excretion within a few weeks of starting treatment (SIRIS et al, 1980; VAN BREUKELEN et al, 1979). However, these studies were small, and uncertainties about the correct dose and schedule, the best route of administration and the methodology of assessing response have made them difficult to interpret.

In our parenteral study APD was able, in the absence of any other systemic treatment for breast cancer, to halt the metastatic destruction of bone. Four patients showed radiological evidence of bone healing, while 11 had stable disease. There was also a reduction in pain score and increased mobility. Symptomatic response was occasionally dramatic, and in some cases osteolytic destruction was inhibited for many months. Toxicity was minimal, the only consistently reported side effect in all studies to date being transient fever.

Inhibition of new bone metastases had previously been noted in both animal and human studies, but none had reported radiological improvement in existing metastatic bone disease. The bisphosphonates possess no cytotoxic or immunosuppressive activity, so these observations need an alternative explanation. Perhaps the specific inhibition of bone resorption reverses the pronounced efflux of calcium from the skeleton, while continuing osteoblast activity permits new bone formation to occur and to appear as sclerosis on plain radiographs. Our results have subsequently been confirmed in a similar study (MORTON et al, 1988).

A fairly consistent early biochemical response was seen, with reduced levels of both serum and urinary calcium. In some patients however osteolysis appeared to become resistant to APD, with a rise in urinary calcium excretion and progressive lysis on X-ray. This may reflect osteolytic mechanisms which are independent of osteoclast activation and/or either tachyphylaxis or falling bone uptake of APD. Interestingly, the initial rate of bone resorption, as measured by urinary calcium excretion, was highest in patients with progressive disease.

Inhibition of bone resorption is not uniform on this parenteral schedule of APD, with the nadir in serum calcium and urinary calcium excretion occurring six days after administration. However, a fortnightly schedule was convenient for outpatient treatment. Oral APD would be more convenient and might achieve a more complete and continuous inhibition of bone resorption; but, because oral absorption of all bisphosphonates is low and variable (0–5%), high doses are necessary, with the risk of gastrointestinal irritation.

The purpose of an effervescent formulation of APD was to avoid high local concentrations in the mouth, oesophagus and stomach. The results of the phase I study showed that effective inhibition of osteolysis was achieved at doses which were well tolerated. Urinary calcium excretion fell to normal even at the lowest dose tested (150 mg daily). The data are insufficient to determine whether this dose is adequate for long-term inhibition of osteolysis, but they do suggest that doses lower than 150 mg daily should be tested before embarking on studies of long-term administration.

Although APD is effective in inhibiting bone resorption secondary to advanced breast cancer, its place in management is most likely to be in conjunction with systemic anticancer therapy. In both our studies extraskeletal progression was common, presumably because APD lacks specific anticancer activity. Whether this influenced the development of bone marrow infiltration and spinal cord compression through intramedullary and epidural extension is speculative, but the incidence of these complications was higher than would have been expected.

To date, only two randomised studies of bisphosphonates in conjunction with systemic therapy have been reported. In the first, ELOMAA et al (1985) randomly assigned 34 patients with progressive bone metastases from breast cancer to receive oral clodronate or placebo in addition to systemic therapy. Analgesic and radiotherapy requirements were reduced in the bisphosphonate-treated group, and the complication rate, number of new bone lesions and progression in existing sites were also less. More recently, a second, much larger study using oral pamidronate (VAN HOLTEN-VERZANTVOORT et al, 1987) reported that the complication rate from skeletal involvement and the number of new bone metastases was significantly less in the pamidronate-treated group.

Conclusions

Many questions persist regarding the use of bisphosphonates. The optimum dose, schedule and route of administration remain unknown, as do their mechanisms of action and long-term effects on the normal skeleton. Studies are under way both to answer these questions and to assess the contribution of bisphosphonates to systemic therapy. The results will help to determine the value of this potentially exciting new development in the management of advanced breast cancer.

References

ADAMI, S., BHALLA, A. K., DORIZZO, R. et al (1987) The acute-phase response after bisphosphonate administration. *Calcif. Tissue Int. 41*, 326–331.

BODY, J. J., POT, M., BORKOWSKI, A. et al (1987) Dose/response study of aminohydroxypropylidene bisphosphonate in tumor-associated hypercalcemia. *Am. J. Med. 82*, 957–963.

COLEMAN, R. E. and RUBENS, R. D. (1987) 3(amino-1,1-hydroxypropylidene) bisphosphonate (APD) for hypercalcaemia of breast cancer. *Br. J. Cancer 56*, 465–469.

COLEMAN, R. E. and RUBENS, R. D. (1990) APD for the treatment of hypercalcaemia of malignancy (HOM): a comparison of different doses and schedules of administration. *Br. J. Cancer* (in press).

COLEMAN, R. E., WOLL, P. J., MILES, M. et al (1988) Treatment of bone metastases from breast cancer with (3-amino-1-hydroxy-propylidene)-1,1-bisphosphonate (APD). *Br. J. Cancer 58*, 621–625.

COLEMAN, R. E., WOLL, P. J. and RUBENS, R. D. (1990) A phase I/II evaluation of a novel oral formulation of APD for the treatment of bone metastases. *Br. J. Cancer* (in press).

ELOMAA, I., BLOMQUIST, C. and PORKKA, L. (1985) Diphosphonates for osteolytic bone metastases. *Lancet i*, 1155–1156.

FLEISCH, H. (1988) Bisphosphonates: A new class of drugs in bone disease and calcium metabolism. In: *Handbook of Experimental Pharmacology,* Vol. 83, P. F. Baker (Ed.), p. 441. Springer, Berlin/Heidelberg.

GARATTINI, S., GUAITANI, A. and MANTOVANI, A. (1987) Effect of etidronate disodium on the interactions between malignancy and bone. *Am. J. Med. 82* (Suppl. 2A), 29–33.

MORTON, A. R., CANTRILL, J. A., PILLAI, G. V. et al (1988) Sclerosis of lytic bone metastases after disodium aminohydroxypropylidene bisphosphonate in patients with breast carcinoma. *Br. Med. J. 297,* 772–773.

SIRIS, E. S., SHERMAN, W. H., BAQUIRAN, D. C. et al (1980) Effects of dichloromethylene diphosphonate on skeletal mobilization of calcium in multiple myeloma. *N. Engl. J. Med. 302,* 310–315.

SLEEBOOM, H. P., BIJVOET, O. L. M., VAN OOSTEROM, A. T. et al (1983) Comparison of intravenous (3 amino-1-hydroxypropylidene)-1,1-bisphosphonate and volume repletion in tumour-induced hypercalcaemia. *Lancet ii,* 239–243.

THIÉBAUD, D., JAEGER, P., JACQUET, A. F. et al (1988) Dose response in the treatment of hypercalcemia of malignancy by a single infusion of the bisphosphonate AHPrBP (APD). *J. Clin. Oncol. 6,* 762–768.

VAN BREUKELEN, F. J. M., BIJVOET, O. L. M. and OOSTEROM, A. T. (1979) Inhibition of osteolytic bone lesions by (3-amino, 1-hydroxypropylidene)-1,1-bisphosphonate (APD). *Lancet i,* 803–805.

VAN HOLTEN-VERZANTVOORT, A., BIJVOET, O. L. M., CLETON, F. J. et al (1987) Reduced morbidity from skeletal metastases in breast cancer patients during long-term bisphosphonate (APD) treatment. *Lancet ii,* 983–985.

Discussion

Dr S. H. RALSTON (Edinburgh): In your experience is oral or intravenous APD better tolerated by patients?

COLEMAN: There is little if any toxicity associated with intravenous therapy, whereas oral therapy can sometimes be difficult. Choice of therapy depends on whether you want chronic suppression of bone resorption or an intermittent effect on bone cell activity.

Dr J. P. ARMAND (Villejuif): What is your preferred method for evaluating bone – CAT scan, bone density or something else?

COLEMAN: I think at the moment we have to rely on the plain radiograph.

Pamidronate (APD) treatment of skeletal metastases from breast cancer

D. J. Dodwell[1]; A. Howell[1] (speaker), A. Morton[1], P. T. Daley-Yates[2] and C. R. Hoggarth[2]

[1]Department of Medical Oncology, Christie Hospital, Manchester, and
[2]Department of Pharmacy, University of Manchester, UK

Summary

The antitumour action, toxicity and biochemical effects of both intravenous and enteric-coated oral pamidronate have been evaluated in two phase I/II trials in patients with bone metastases from breast cancer.

In the intravenous trial, 22 assessable patients with progressive bone metastases were treated with 30 mg pamidronate weekly for four weeks, and thereafter fortnightly for six months or until disease progression. Response, as defined by sclerosis of previous lytic metastases, occurred in four patients, and an additional seven patients achieved stable disease. There was a significant reduction in calcium excretion and improved control of pain. In addition, the pharmacokinetics of pamidronate were studied in five patients.

In the oral study, 16 women with progressive bone metastases and evidence of active bone resorption were given enteric-coated pamidronate 150 mg to 600 mg daily. Urinary calcium/creatinine ratios fell from a mean of 0.81 at entry to 0.2 after treatment.

There were no significant differences in efficacy between treatment groups. Oral pamidronate is well tolerated at doses of 300 mg or less, and daily doses of 150 mg or more reduce calcium excretion as effectively as 30 mg intravenously once weekly.

Introduction

As many as 84% of patients with breast cancer develop bone metastases (CADMAN and BERTINO, 1976). Currently available treatments – endocrine therapy, cytotoxic drugs and radiotherapy to sites of painful lesions – are useful for controlling progression of the disease, but benefit is often transitory, and many patients show continued bone destruction with associated pain, immobility, pathological fracture and hypercalcaemia. There is thus a pressing need for more effective agents to reduce the considerable morbidity associated with bone metastases.

The bisphosphonates are enzyme-resistant analogues of pyrophosphate, the naturally occurring inhibitor of bone mineralisation. They bind to hydroxyapatite crystals, inhibit osteoclast function and slow the rate of osteoclast-mediated bone resorption (FLEISCH, 1983). They are the treatment of choice for the hypercalcaemia of malignancy, a syndrome characterised almost invariably by excessive bone resorption and, when used in combination with fluid replacement, are over 90% effective in restoring normocalcaemia (MORTON et al, 1988a; JUNG et al, 1981). One placebo-controlled study (VAN HOLTEN-VERZANT-VOORT et al, 1987), using oral pamidronate in combination with standard treatment, showed a reduced incidence of pathological fracture, hypercalcaemia and need for radiotherapy at sites of painful bone lesions in the treated group. There are also favourable reports (MORTON et al, 1988b; COLEMAN et al, 1988) which indicate that intravenous pamidronate given as fortnightly infusions can heal lytic metastases in approximately 25% of patients, and stabilise disease in a further 25%. This report updates our previous study (MORTON et al, 1988b) using intravenous pamidronate and summarises data on an oral enteric-coated formulation (DODWELL and HOWELL, 1990). There is a lack of pharmacokinetic information on intravenous pamidronate, and we have therefore studied its pharmacokinetics in a small group of patients.

Study 1: Intravenous pamidronate in patients with breast cancer metastatic to bone

Methods

Twenty-two assessable female patients with histologically-proven advanced breast cancer were studied. All had purely skeletal metastases, which had progressed on at least one form of endocrine or cytotoxic therapy. In 13 patients endocrine therapy was continued despite disease progression, in order to prevent confusion with a possible endocrine withdrawal response; the remaining nine patients received no other form of antitumour therapy.

After baseline radiology, biochemical assessment, and estimation of urinary hydroxyproline and calcium excretion, all patients were given weekly infusions of 30 mg pamidronate in 500 ml normal saline for four weeks, and then fortnightly thereafter for a total of six months or until disease progression. At each visit patients were asked about their use of analgesics and any unpleasant effects of treatment, and completed a linear analogue pain score and symptom questionnaire of the Rotterdam Check List type (DE HAES et al, 1983). X-rays were repeated at three-monthly intervals. Partial response in bone was defined as sclerosis of previously lytic lesions without the development of new lesions. 'No change' indicated no increase or decrease in the radiological extent of disease for at least six months.

Results

One patient was hypercalcaemic at entry to the study; her serum calcium fell to the normal range during the first two weeks of treatment and remained normal thereafter, in common with all other patients. The fasting urinary calcium/creatinine ratio (as an index of calcium excretion) was elevated (>0.4 mmol/mmol) in 16 patients at entry. This parameter fell significantly ($P<0.001$) after the first infusion of pamidronate, indicating prompt inhibition of bone resorption; there was a tendency for those who responded radiologically to have the lowest ratios. This ratio remained low in all patients except for those whose disease progressed in bone (Fig. 1). The mean urinary hydroxyproline/cre-

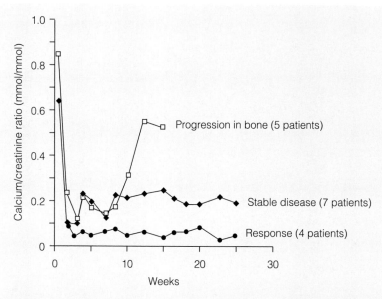

Fig. 1. Calcium/creatinine ratios (mmol/mmol) in 16 patients treated with intravenous pamidronate who had an elevated ratio at start of therapy.

atinine ratio did not change significantly during the study (Fig. 2). The alkaline phosphatase was elevated in most patients at entry, and treatment did not cause any significant change in this value.

The tumour markers CEA (carcinoembryonic antigen) and CA-15.3 were assayed at the time of entry and at monthly intervals thereafter. The levels fell in parallel in three patients (one of whom had a partial response radiologically and one who showed 'no change'), remained essentially unaltered in eight patients and rose in the remaining 11 patients.

Pain scores assessed by linear analogue scales fell significantly ($P < 0.01$) during treatment (Fig. 3), but did not necessarily correlate with radiological or biochemical improvement, so that a placebo effect cannot be excluded. Analysis of analgesic requirements during the course of the study did, however, show a statistically significant reduction ($P < 0.01$) in analgesic usage. Symptoms other than pain, as detailed on the Rotterdam Symptom Check List, also showed improvement ($P < 0.05$), but failed to correlate with more objective assessments of disease regression.

There was radiological evidence of sclerosis of lytic metastases in four patients, whose durations of response were 11, 12, 14 and 17 months. There was no change – with a minimum duration of six months to qualify for this category – in a further seven patients (duration 8–14 months, median nine months). Overall time to progression in these 11 patients is shown in Figure 4. As with most forms of systemic anticancer therapy, patients responding or with stable disease after pamidronate survived significantly longer than those with progressive disease (Fig. 5). Eleven patients did not complete the six-month study

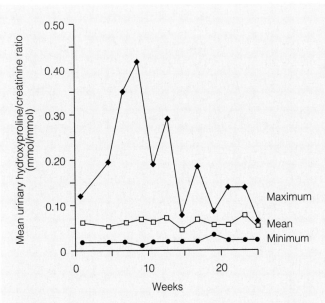

Fig. 2. Urinary excretion of hydroxyproline during and after pamidronate therapy. All patients were fasted overnight and measurements were made on the second morning sample of urine.

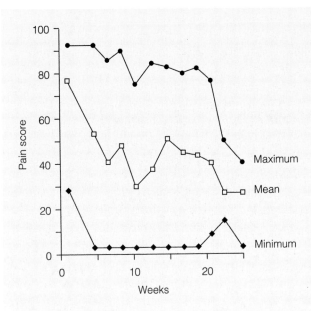

Fig. 3. The effect of intravenous pamidronate on mean pain score, assessed using a 10 cm linear analogue scale.

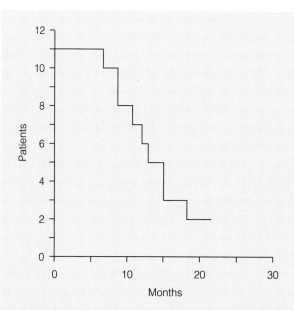

Fig. 4. Time to progression in patients achieving a response (four patients) or with stable disease (no change for a minimum of six months, seven patients) after intravenous pamidronate.

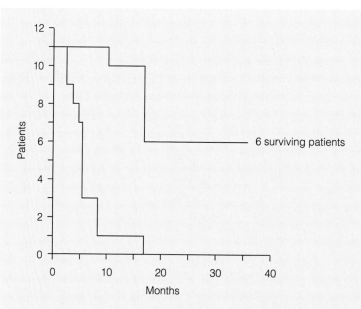

Fig. 5. Survival of patients receiving intravenous pamidronate whose disease regressed or did not change for a minimum of six months (top line), compared with those whose disease progressed within 6 months (bottom line). Median survival for responders 17 months; median survival for progressors 6 months: *P* <0.001.

period because they had progressive disease; in five of them, progression occurred in bone and was associated with elevation of the urinary calcium/creatinine ratio (Fig. 1).

All patients tolerated their infusions well, with no side effects other than a mild, asymptomatic pyrexia in a small number of cases. Thrombophlebitis did not occur, but four patients noted a transient increase in pain after the first dose of pamidronate.

Study 2: Oral pamidronate in women with progressive bone metastases from breast cancer – a phase I/II study

Methods

Sixteen women with breast cancer metastatic to bone (Table I) were treated with enteric-coated pamidronate (Ciba-Geigy). Each group of four patients received 150, 300, 450, or 600 mg daily for four weeks. All had bone metastases confirmed by isotope scintigraphy and plain radiology, and evidence of raised calcium excretion as measured by the calcium/creatinine ratio in fasting urine samples. All had received at least one form of endocrine treatment, and four had also received cytotoxic therapy. Endocrine treatment was continued, even when disease progressed, to prevent confusing response to pamidronate

Table I. Characteristics of patients treated with oral pamidronate.

Patient	Age (years)	Dose (mg/day)	Disease-free interval (months)	Type of bone metastases	Previous treatments	Duration of current endocrine treatment (months)
1	57	150	108	Mixed	Both	N/A
2	51	150	13	Lytic	ET	10
3	51	150	28	Mixed	ET	23
4	42	150	22	Lytic	Both	5
5	49	300	84	Lytic	ET	N/A
6	78	300	120	Lytic	ET	46
7	41	300	26	Mixed	ET	5
8	51	300	20	Lytic	ET	8
9	57	450	70	Mixed	Both	11
10	56	450	0	Mixed	ET	14
11	76	450	0	Mixed	ET	11
12	64	450	11	Mixed	ET	14
13	54	600	15	Mixed	Both	N/A
14	48	600	21	Lytic	ET	14
15	46	600	28	Mixed	ET	N/A
16	52	600	31	Mixed	ET	16

ET   = endocrine therapy
Both = cytotoxic and endocrine therapy
N/A = not applicable

with a possible hormone withdrawal response. During the first month of therapy the patients were seen weekly, thereafter at monthly intervals. At each attendance a fasting urine sample was analysed for calcium and creatinine, serum biochemistry and haematology were performed, and patients were interviewed about their use of analgesics and any unpleasant effects of treatment. At the end of four weeks, and in the absence of adverse effects, patients continued to take 300 mg pamidronate daily. The values of the calcium/creatinine ratio in all patients were subjected to a two-way analysis of variance to study differences between initial values and those after treatment, and also to determine whether there was a significant difference between treatment groups.

Results

The initial urinary calcium/creatinine ratios ranged from 0.42 to 2.1 (mean 0.8 mmol/mmol), and there were no significant differences in the initial values between the four groups of patients. There was a significant fall in calcium excretion at all doses of pamidronate; this occurred within one week of treatment and tended to be maximal by three weeks (Figs 6 and 7). In patients on 150 mg daily the mean ratio fell from 0.65 (range 0.57–0.72) before treatment to 0.13 (range 0.02–0.19) after three weeks. Mean values at entry for patients on 300, 450 and 600 mg were 1.18 (range 0.72–2.1), 0.76 (range 0.42–1.5) and 0.63 (range 0.52–0.82) respectively; after treatment these fell to 0.11 (range

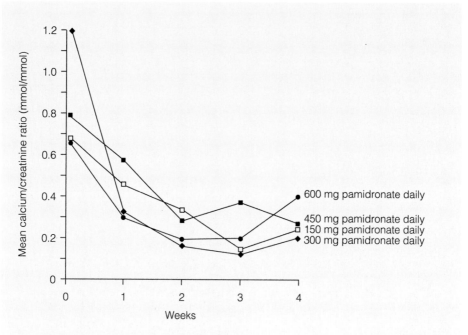

Fig. 6. Effect of oral enteric-coated pamidronate at various doses on mean urinary calcium/creatinine ratios. Each line is the mean value from four patients receiving the specified daily dose of pamidronate.

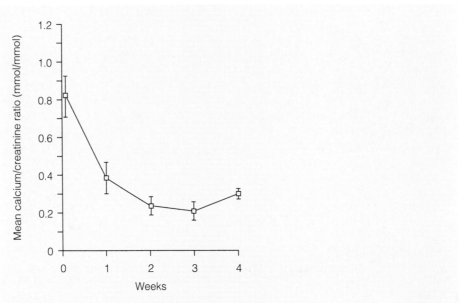

Fig. 7. Urinary calcium/creatinine ratios in all patients treated with oral pamidronate (*n* = 16).

0.05–0.18), 0.37 (range 0.14–0.68) and 0.17 (range 0.06–0.25). There was no significant difference in the calcium/creatinine ratio between the four groups. The data from each group were combined to give the overall result shown in Figure 7. There was a significant fall in the ratio after one week ($P<0.01$) and a highly significant fall after three weeks. The median subsequent follow-up time was 15 weeks (range 7–21 weeks). In twelve patients the calcium/creatinine ratio remained low, but in four there was progression of disease in bone despite treatment, and a rise of the mean ratio to the pretreatment level (Fig. 8). In the intravenous study 16 of the 22 patients had evidence of elevated calcium excretion at entry. In this group the mean calcium/creatinine ratio fell from 0.85 (range 0.44–1.4) to a minimum of 0.19 (range 0.02–0.67) after treatment with pamidronate. There was no significant difference in the rate of fall of the ratio in this group, compared to the 16 patients treated with the oral preparation (Fig. 9).

At a median follow-up of 15 weeks there was no discernible effect on mean pain scores in this study, though certain patients reported substantial improvement. Similarly, symptoms other than pain, as assessed by the Rotterdam Symptom Check List, also appear to be unaffected by oral pamidronate. No radiological responses have been seen. Seven patients have suffered disease progression – four in bone and three at other sites. Follow-up is too short to permit any meaningful comment on the other nine patients.

There was no gastrointestinal toxicity at doses of 150 mg and 300 mg daily. At 450 mg daily one out of four patients experienced WHO grade 1 nausea and abdominal pain for eight days, one week after starting treatment. Reducing

69

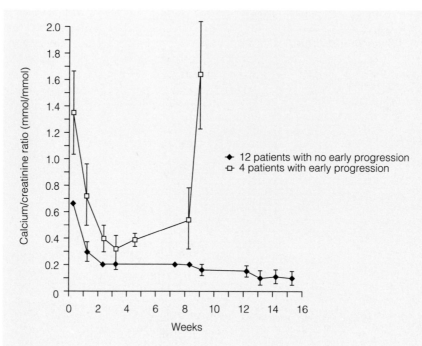

Fig. 8. Urinary calcium/creatinine ratios in patients who progressed early in bone ($n = 4$) compared with those who did not ($n = 12$).

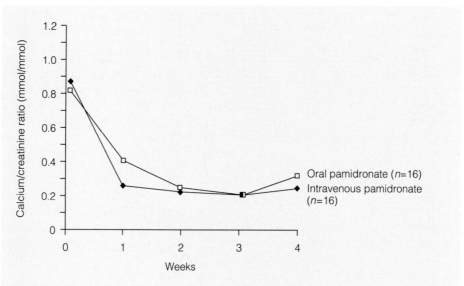

Fig. 9. Comparison between the urinary calcium/creatinine ratios of patients treated with oral enteric-coated pamidronate and those receiving intravenous pamidronate.

the dose to 300 mg abolished this. At 600 mg daily one out of four patients required a reduction in dose because of similar gastrointestinal toxicity, but tolerated 300 mg daily without further problems. Oral ulceration was not seen, and there was no haematological toxicity at any dosage level. Two patients on 600 mg daily developed asymptomatic hypocalcaemia (corrected calcium 2.08–2.17 mmol/l; normal range 2.2–2.65 mmol/l) one week after starting treatment; this persisted for one week in one patient and for two weeks in the other.

Study 3: The pharmacokinetics of intravenous pamidronate

Methods

To date we have studied the pharmacokinetics of pamidronate in five patients with hypercalcaemia of malignancy. Each received 60 mg pamidronate as the anhydrous disodium salt, dissolved in 500 ml of normal saline, by intravenous infusion over eight or 24 hours.

Blood (5 ml) was collected in lithium heparin tubes at 15 minutes, 30 minutes, one hour, two hours, four hours, eight hours and 24 hours where appropriate after the start of the infusion, the last sample being taken immediately before the end of infusion. Within a few minutes of collection the blood was centrifuged to separate the plasma, which was stored at –20°C prior to analysis for pamidronate. The infusion was started after emptying the bladder, and the urine was collected for the following 24 hours, the time and volume being recorded and a 20 ml aliquot removed and stored at –20°C prior to analysis.

Pamidronate was analysed according to the method of DALEY-YATES et al (1989), which is similar for both plasma and urine samples. An internal standard (1-hydroxy-5-aminopentylidene-1,1-bisphosphonate) is first added to the sample, followed by calcium chloride to cause precipitation of the bisphosphonates as their calcium salts. After centrifugation the precipitate is redissolved in acetic acid, and the samples are then separated by high performance ion chromatography, using an on-line two-stage post-column reaction. The bisphosphonates are oxidised to orthophosphate by the addition of ammonium persulphate, and then mixed with a molybdenum-ascorbate reagent to yield a phosphomolybdate chromophore detectable at 820 nm. The detection limit is 10 ng/ml.

Results

Figure 10 shows the plasma concentration/time profile and urine excretion data for a typical patient following infusion of 60 mg pamidronate over eight hours. Analysis of the plasma concentration data during the infusion, by non-linear least squares regression, revealed an initial half-life of approximately 30 minutes. The terminal half-life of the drug is very long, however, and can only be estimated from the urinary excretion rate against time plot – a value of over two years was calculated from the 24 hour infusion data. Despite this, all patients had plasma concentrations of pamidronate approaching a plateau within the first few hours of infusion. During the infusion period approximately 25% of the dose appeared in the urine; after the infusion little additional

71

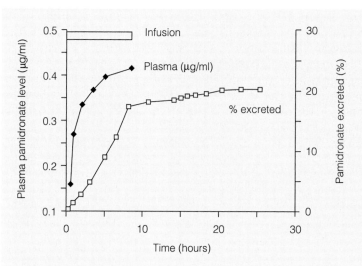

Fig. 10. Plasma and urinary pharmacokinetics of pamidronate in a patient receiving 60 mg infused over eight hours in 500 ml normal saline.

drug was excreted. The mean total clearance (calculated from the infusion rate divided by the plasma concentration at the end of the infusion) of pamidronate for the five subjects was 223 ml/min (range 144–298 ml/min). The mean renal clearance (calculated from the amount excreted during the infusion divided by the corresponding plasma AUC) was 49.9 ml/min (range 31.4–68.6 ml/min), leaving a non-renal clearance for pamidronate of 173 ml/min. Since this drug is not known to be metabolised the clearance may be predominantly by uptake into the skeleton, which over the period of this study appears to act as a sink for pamidronate.

Conclusions

These preliminary data show that pamidronate has a very high clearance, due predominantly to retention in the skeleton, and partly to renal clearance. Most of the drug is cleared from the plasma before distribution equilibrium is achieved, resulting in the rapid attainment of an apparent steady-state plasma concentration within a few hours from the start of intravenous infusion. However, the initial short half-life soon gives way to a prolonged elimination phase which probably reflects slow release of pamidronate from deep tissue compartments such as bone.

Discussion (all three studies)

Used in conjunction with other systemic treatments for advanced breast cancer, bisphosphonates have been shown to reduce pain, and the frequency of hypercalcaemia and pathological fracture (VAN HOLTEN-VERZANTVOORT et al,

1987; ELOMAA et al, 1983). They are also highly effective in controlling the hypercalcaemia of malignancy (MORTON et al, 1988a). These studies pose the question whether giving bisphosphonates alone would prevent osteoclast-mediated bone resorption in women with metastases confined to bone (MORTON et al, 1988b). Since tumour products are known to stimulate osteoblast function (PFEILSCHIFTER et al, 1987; CENTRELLA et al, 1987) we hypothesised that new bone might be stimulated to replace tumour when osteoclast-mediated bone destruction was inhibited.

The dose of pamidronate used in the intravenous study was based on that known to control most cases of hypercalcaemia (COLEMAN and RUBENS, 1987). In previous reports of this study (MORTON et al, 1988b) we assessed 16 patients: four had a partial remission as judged by sclerosis of previously lytic lesions, four showed no progression of disease for at least six months, while eight had progressive disease. We regard 'no change' for six months as a response to treatment, since we have reported that the survival of such patients is equivalent to those who have a partial remission (HOWELL et al, 1988). In this updated report the response rate remains the same (11/22: 50%) in a larger group of patients. Resclerosis of lytic metastases and disease stabilisation using bisphosphonates alone have now been confirmed by other groups (COLEMAN et al, 1988; COLEMAN, 1990; LIPTON et al, 1990).

Treatment was stopped after six months, according to the protocol. Despite this, responses continued for a further eight months, and might have continued longer if we had maintained the fortnightly infusions. Non-responders to pamidronate in this study survived a median of six months only, suggesting aggressive disease. The median survival of responders has not yet been reached but is in excess of 18 months: this suggests that pamidronate may be more effective in women with relatively slowly progressive bone disease (all had progressive bone disease at the start of treatment). It is too early to comment on the responses to oral pamidronate.

In animal studies, and in patients with osteoporosis given adequate doses of pamidronate, the calcium/creatinine ratio falls uniformly, suggesting that normal osteoclasts are not resistant to bisphosphonates. In both our studies there were initial falls in calcium excretion, and in responders it remained low until progression (Fig. 1); in women with progressive disease in bone, calcium excretion rose soon after the initial fall. The reason for this initial fall and subsequent rise is not clear: perhaps tumour products which stimulate osteoclast function have sufficient potency to overcome the inhibitory effect of pamidronate on these cells. This hypothesis can be tested either by performing dose-response studies with pamidronate (LIPTON et al, 1990) or by using more potent bisphosphonates.

We have seen little change in serum levels of alkaline phosphatase or osteocalcin, suggesting that pamidronate has no effect on osteoblast activity. Surprisingly there was no change in hydroxyproline excretion, either because urinary levels were largely a reflection of extraskeletal collagen breakdown, or because there was no inhibition of osteoblast or tumour-cell collagenase production during pamidronate treatment.

No clinically relevant toxic effects were seen with intravenous pamidronate. At oral doses above 300 mg daily gastrointestinal disturbances became a problem. However, in the small number of patients studied, the ability of pamidronate to reduce calcium excretion was not increased by higher doses, so such doses may not be necessary.

Assuming that 1% of the oral formulation is absorbed, at least 30 mg will be available to bone over a two-week period if 300 mg is given daily – similar to 30 mg intravenously every two weeks. Our pharmacokinetic studies show that less than half of the administered dose is excreted over 24 hours, consistent with data indicating a half-life for pamidronate in bone of more than six months (WINGEN and SCHMÄHL, 1987). However, in hypercalcaemia the effectiveness of a single infusion in maintaining a normal serum calcium is only 2–3 weeks; in normocalcaemic patients with bone metastases a single dose of pamidronate intravenously lowers the urinary calcium for 2–6 weeks. The relatively short duration of anti-osteoclast activity must indicate that pamidronate, when retained within the body for long periods, is not readily available to the osteoclast. Thus daily oral therapy may be superior to intermittent infusion for osteoclast inhibition. Confirmation of this hypothesis requires further data on the clinical activity and pharmacokinetics of oral pamidronate.

Acknowledgement

We would like to thank Ciba-Geigy Pharmaceuticals for supplies of pamidronate and for financial support.

References

CADMAN, E. and BERTINO, J. R. (1976) Chemotherapy of skeletal metastases. *Int. J. Radiat. Oncol. Biol. Phys. 1,* 1211–1215.

CENTRELLA, M., McCARTHY, T. L. and CANALIS, E. (1987) Transforming growth factor β is a bifunctional regulator of replication and collagen synthesis in osteoblast-enriched cell cultures from fetal rat bone. *J. Biol. Chem. 262,* 2869–2874.

COLEMAN, R. E. (1990) Pamidronate (APD) treatment of bone metastases from breast cancer. In: *The Management of Bone Metastases and Hypercalcaemia by Osteoclast Inhibition,* R. D. Rubens (Ed.), pp. 52–61. Hogrefe and Huber, Toronto/Lewiston N.Y./Bern/Göttingen/Stuttgart.

COLEMAN, R. E. and RUBENS, R. D. (1987) Treatment of hypercalcaemia secondary to advanced breast cancer with 3-(amino-1,1-hydroxypropylidene) bisphosphonate (APD). *Br. J. Cancer 56,* 465–469.

COLEMAN, R. E., WOLL, P. J., MILES, M. et al (1988) 3-amino-1,1-hydroxypropylidene bisphosphonate (APD) for the treatment of bone metastases from breast cancer. *Br. J. Cancer 58,* 621–625.

DALEY-YATES, P. T., GIFFORD, L. A. and HOGGARTH, C. R. (1989) Assay of 1-hydroxy-3-aminopropylidene-1,1-bisphosphonate, and related bisphosphonates, in human urine and plasma by high performance ion chromatography. *J. Chromatogr. 490,* 329–338.

DE HAES, J., PRUYN, J. F. A. and VAN KNIPPENBERG, F. C. E. (1983) Klachtenlijst voor kankerpatienten. Eerste evaringen. *Ned. Tijdschr. Psychol. 38,* 403–422.

DODWELL, D. J. and HOWELL, A. (1990) Reduction in calcium excretion in women with breast cancer and bone metastases using the oral bisphosphonate pamidronate. *Br. J. Cancer,* in press.

ELOMAA, I., BLOMQUIST, C., GROHN, P. et al (1983) Long-term controlled trial with diphosphonate in patients with osteolytic bone metastases. *Lancet i,* 146–148.

FLEISCH, H. (1983) Bisphosphonates, mechanisms of action and clinical applications. In: *Bone and Mineral Research, Annual 1,* W. A. Peck (Ed.), pp. 319–357. Excerpta Medica, Amsterdam.

Howell, A., Mackintosh, J., Jones, M. et al (1988) The definition of the 'no change' category in patients treated with endocrine therapy and chemotherapy for advanced carcinoma of the breast. *Eur. J. Cancer Clin. Oncol. 24*, 1567–1572.

Jung, A., van Ouwenaller, C., Chantraine, A. et al (1981) Parenteral diphosphonates for treating malignant hypercalcaemia. *Cancer 48*, 1922–1925.

Lipton, A., Harvey, H., Givant, E. et al (1990) Disodium pamidronate (APD) – a dose-seeking study in patients with breast and prostate cancer. In: *The Management of Bone Metastases and Hypercalcaemia by Osteoclast Inhibition*, R. D. Rubens (Ed.), pp. 90–100. Hogrefe and Huber, Toronto/Lewiston N.Y./Bern/Göttingen/Stuttgart.

Morton, A. R., Cantrill, J. A., Craig, A. E. et al (1988a) Single dose versus daily intravenous aminohydroxypropylidene bisphosphonate (APD) for the hypercalcaemia of malignancy. *Br. Med. J. 296*, 811–814.

Morton, A. R., Cantrill, J. A., Pillai, G. V. et al (1988b) Sclerosis of lytic bone metastases after disodium aminohydroxypropylidene bisphosphonate (APD) in patients with breast carcinoma. *Br. Med. J. 297*, 772–773.

Pfeilschifter, J., D'Souza, S. M. and Mundy, G. R. (1987) Effects of transforming growth factor beta on osteoblastic osteosarcoma cells. *Endocrinology 121*, 212–218.

van Holten-Verzantvoort, A., Bijvoet, O. L. M., Cleton, F. J. et al (1987) Reduced morbidity from skeletal metastases in breast cancer patients during long-term bisphosphonate (APD) treatment. *Lancet ii*, 983–985.

Wingen, F. and Schmähl, D. (1987) Pharmacokinetics of the osteotropic diphosphonate 3-amino-1-hydroxypropane-1,1-diphosphonic acid in mammals. *Arzneimittelforsch./Drug Res. 37*, 1037–1042.

Discussion

Dr A. Efremidis (Athens): Do you have any information on the estrogen or progesterone receptor status of patients who responded to treatment?

Howell: No. At present our data do not allow us to draw any conclusions.

Use of disodium bisphosphonate (APD) in the treatment of breast cancer and myeloma bone metastases

S. Leyvraz[1], D. Thiébaud[2], V. von Fliedner[3], L. Peyrey[1], P. Cornu[1], S. Thiébaud[4] and P. Burckhardt[2]

Departments of [1]Oncology, [2]Internal Medicine and [4]Radiology, and [3]Ludwig Institute for Cancer Research, University Hospital, Lausanne, Switzerland

Summary

In an open study, 25 patients with breast cancer, 12 with myeloma and one with lymphocytic lymphoma were treated with monthly infusions of APD 60 mg for four months, then every three months until disease progression. All patients had painful, progressive, osteolytic bone metastases from histologically proven disease.

Among the patients with breast cancer there were statistically significant falls in serum and urinary calcium, and in urinary hydroxyproline; eight of the 18 evaluable patients showed radiological evidence of sclerosis, and nine showed symptomatic improvement. Nine of the ten evaluable patients with myeloma showed symptomatic improvement, but in only one was there evidence of sclerosis.

APD appears to be a safe and well tolerated therapy able to relieve bone pain, induce sclerosis and correct serum and urinary calcium levels in a proportion of patients.

Introduction

Bisphosphonates have been of interest to endocrinologists and specialists in calcium and bone pathophysiology for many years. At the beginning of the 1980s oncologists also became interested in bisphosphonates when they were shown to be effective in treating and controlling hypercalcaemia due to malignant disease. The next step was to test bisphosphonates as an adjuvant to oncological therapies when malignant disease involved bone.

We have studied a group of unselected patients with painful, progressive, osteolytic metastases from histologically proven breast cancer or myeloma; in addition, one patient with a low-grade, diffuse, well differentiated lymphocytic lymphoma was included in the myeloma group. The aims of the study were to test the effects of high-dose intravenous APD on bone resorption and on pain, and to assess its long-term tolerability.

Patients and methods

Patients were divided in two groups: those with histologically proven breast cancer, and those with myeloma. Inclusion criteria comprised:
– absence of hypercalcaemia

- no change in oncological treatment
- radiotherapy to be completed before inclusion in the study
- at least two courses of APD, and
- a follow-up period of at least three months.

Biochemical evaluation consisted of monthly serum calcium, phosphate, creatinine, proteins and alkaline phosphatase, together with urinary calcium, phosphate, creatinine and hydroxyproline from a two-hourly morning sample. Subjective evaluation was also undertaken monthly, using a pain analogue scale completed by the patient and a scoring scale completed by the oncologist. Analgesic use and performance status according to ECOG (Eastern Cooperative Oncology Group) were recorded. Plain X-rays of involved areas were taken every three months and reviewed 'blind' by a radiologist. Treatment consisted of 60 mg APD, given as a 24-hour intravenous infusion every month for four months, and then every three months until progression of disease. In the majority of cases treatment was given on an outpatient basis, using a portable pump.

Patient characteristics are summarised in Table I. Twenty-five patients with breast cancer were enrolled, but seven were subsequently ineligible because of early death (less than three months on study), or because they only received one course of APD – reflecting the advanced stage of disease among the treated patients. Thirteen patients with myeloma were included, of whom three subsequently became ineligible for similar reasons.

In the breast cancer group, the median age was 57 years; six patients were less than 49 years old, and premenopausal. Eleven patients in this group started a new oncological treatment at the same time as APD, but this was not changed again during the study; seven patients either received no oncological treatment at all, or did not change hormonal therapy commenced between one and three years previously. This subgroup is presented separately so that the role of APD can be better evaluated.

Table I. Characteristics of patients enrolled in the trial.

	Breast cancer	Myeloma
Entered	25	13
– Eligible and evaluable	18	10
– Ineligible	7	3
Mean age (range)	57 (37–85) years	64 (39–83) years
Oncological treatment		
– None or no change	7	8
– New (at same time as starting APD)	11	2
Number of courses of APD (range)	4 (2–12)	7 (3-10)

Results

The biochemical results for the breast cancer group showed significant falls in serum calcium, urinary calcium and urinary hydroxyproline, suggesting an important reduction in the rate of bone resorption (Table II). For the same group, Table III shows the subjective and radiological results. Symptomatic improvement occurred in half the patients, and lasted between three and 14 months. Radiological evidence of sclerosis appeared in eight cases, but an identical number showed progressive changes. Looking in more detail at the subgroup of patients who received no oncological treatment or no new treatment, four out of seven showed symptomatic improvement, of whom three showed evidence of bone sclerosis on X-rays for between six and 18 months. One of three patients with sclerosis had no symptomatic improvement, however.

In the myeloma group, the criteria for diminution of bone resorption were met in every case, with a rapid fall in urinary calcium and hydroxyproline that levelled out at around 50% of the initial values. Looking at the subjective and radiological results (Table IV) it is clear that these patients did not show the

Table II. Selected biochemical results in patients with breast cancer ($\pm$ s.e. mean).

	Day 0	Day 150	Significance of difference
Serum calcium (mmol/l)	2.51 ($\pm$0.05)	2.40 ($\pm$0.04)	$P < 0.05$
Urinary calcium (μmol/mmol creatinine)	0.70 ($\pm$0.07)	0.40 ($\pm$0.05)	$P < 0.01$
Urinary hydroxyproline (μmol/mmol creatinine)	60.4 ($\pm$8.9)	38.9 ($\pm$5.0)	$P < 0.01$

Table III. Subjective and radiological results among the 18 evaluable patients with breast cancer.

Subjective results	
– Improvement	9 (50%)
– No change	8 (44%)
– Deterioration	1 (6%)
Radiological results	
– Sclerosis	8 (44%)
– No change	2 (12%)
– Progression	8 (44%)

Table IV. Subjective and radiological results among the ten evaluable patients with myeloma. Patient 1 had no pain and was considered inevaluable for subjective response; patient 6 had a low-grade, diffuse, well differentiated lymphocytic lymphoma.

Patient	Oncological treatment	Symptoms	Duration of response (months)	X-ray appearances
1	None	(Inevaluable)	(–)	Sclerosis
2	None	Improvement	18	No change
3	None	Improvement	18	No change
4	None	Improvement	16	No change
5	None	Improvement	10	No change
6	None	Improvement	24	No change
7	Melphalan-Pred*	Improvement	9	(No data)
8	Chlorambucil-Pred**	Improvement	6	No change
9	Melphalan-Pred	Improvement	12	No change
10	Melphalan	No change	–	No change

* Melphalan and prednisone for the previous three months
** Chlorambucil and prednisone for the previous three years

same pattern of response as those with breast cancer. Eight showed a dramatic improvement in symptoms, which lasted between six and 24 months; one patient had no pain and was considered inevaluable for symptomatic response. On the other hand, except for one patient who developed sclerosis of lytic lesions, no radiological changes were observed. There was no difference in response between those patients receiving oncological treatment and those not receiving it.

Side effects in both groups were minor. Two patients developed superficial phlebitis and one a transient fever. No haematological or renal changes were recorded.

Conclusions

APD, given intravenously in high dosage on a monthly basis, proved a safe and well tolerated therapy. It produced a significant reduction in bone resorption, as shown by the fall in serum and urinary calcium levels, and by the radiological evidence of bone sclerosis in eight breast cancer patients. Symptomatic improvement occurred in half the patients with breast cancer and in nine out of ten of those with myeloma.

Further reading

COLEMAN, R.E., WOLL, P.J., MILES, M. et al (1988) Treatment of bone metastases from breast cancer with (3-amino-1-hydroxypropylidene)-1, 1-bisphosphonate (APD). *Br. J. Cancer 58,* 621–625.

DELMAS, P. D., CHARHON, S., CHAPUY, M. C. et al (1982) Long-term effects of dichloromethylene diphosphonate (C12 MDP) on skeletal lesions in multiple myeloma. *Metab. Bone Dis. Rel. Res. 4*, 163–168.

FLEISCH, H. (1987) Bisphosphonates – history and experimental basis. *Bone 8* (Suppl. 1), 23–28.

THIÉBAUD, D., JAEGER, P., JACQUET, A. F. et al (1986) A single-day treatment of tumor-induced hypercalcemia by intravenous aminohydroxypropylidene bisphosphonate. *J. Bone Min. Res. 1*, 555–562.

THIÉBAUD, D., JAEGER, P., GOBELET, C. et al (1988) A single infusion of bisphosphonate AHPrBP (APD) as treatment of Paget's disease of bone. *Am. J. Med. 85*, 207–212.

Discussion

Dr J. P. ARMAND (Villejuif): I found it difficult in your study to determine the extent of bone metastases. To answer the question 'Who are the good responders?' we need far more detailed patient profiles, both clinically and in terms of laboratory data, especially receptor status.

LEYVRAZ: We do in fact have most of the data you mention – previous chemotherapy, bone involvement and so on – but there was too much to show today. I agree that receptor status may be an important prognostic factor for response to APD in breast cancer patients.

Subjective and metabolic effects of aminohydroxypropylidene bisphosphonate (APD) in patients with advanced cancer of the prostate – preliminary report

N. W. Clarke[1], J. McClure[2] and N. J. R. George[1]

[1]Department of Urology, University Hospital of South Manchester, and
[2]Department of Histopathology, University of Manchester, UK

Summary

Twenty-six patients with sclerotic bone metastases from prostatic cancer were treated with APD (30 mg/500 ml NaCl over three hours) weekly for four weeks, then twice monthly for five months. Bone scans, X-rays and double tetracycline-labelled iliac crest biopsies were undertaken before and after treatment. Bone turnover was monitored monthly using fasting morning urinary hydroxyproline/creatinine ratios and fasting urine calcium excretion (Ca_E), serum alkaline phosphatase and osteocalcin. Pain and mobility scores were assigned at each visit.

Results showed a diminished hydroxyproline/creatinine ratio in 16 patients at one month. Falls were sustained in 13 patients at three months and 12 patients at six months. Nine patients had increased levels at six months (all with increasing tumour load) and four patients died whilst undergoing treatment. Serial values for Ca_E showed a significant and sustained fall on treatment, and tumour-free iliac crest biopsies showed falls in osteoid surface and volume, and in eroded surface ($P < 0.02$) following treatment. Bone volume and mineralisation rate were also significantly lowered at this dosage ($P < 0.01$ and < 0.001 respectively). Of 18 patients with pain, ten experienced some relief with correspondingly improved mobility and decreased analgesic requirement.

Introduction

Prostatic cancer is the fourth most common cause of death from malignant disease in Britain (Tate et al, 1979), and its predilection to metastasise to bone is well documented (Jacobs, 1983). Such metastases usually increase morbidity as well as mortality (Whitmore, 1956). This study assesses the role of the bisphosphonate APD in patients with advanced prostatic cancer and bone metastases, with particular reference to its efficacy in controlling disturbed metabolic function in bone, and hence its ability to minimise the related morbidity.

Patients and methods

Over an 18-month period 26 patients (mean age 74.1 years, range 62–87) were treated with APD. All had scintigraphic evidence of bone metastases, and all had undergone hormone manipulation at least six months previously. (The mean period following hormone manipulation was 24.4 months.) Skeletal scintigraphy and radiology were undertaken six months before, immediately before and following completion of treatment. Patients received intravenous APD 30 mg over three hours weekly for four weeks, and then twice monthly for five months. Analogue pain and Karnofsky mobility scores were assigned at each visit and metabolic bone activity was assessed each month using serum alkaline phosphatase and osteocalcin, together with fasting morning urinary hydroxyproline/creatinine ratios and urinary calcium excretion. Tumour progression was monitored by acid phosphatase. After initial double tetracycline labelling, transiliac trephine bone biopsies were taken before and after treatment and undecalcified sections were analysed using standard histomorphometric techniques.

Results

Infusions were well tolerated, without appreciable side effects. Four patients died during treatment, and one was too ill to continue after five months.
The effects of treatment as assessed by skeletal scintigraphy are shown in Figure 1. Seventeen patients showed deterioration on bone scans prior to treatment, as judged by increasing size and/or number of metastases on con-

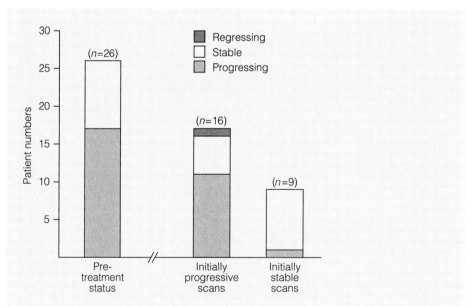

Fig. 1. The bone scan status of 26 patients before and after treatment with APD, as assessed by skeletal scintigraphy. The pretreatment column ($n = 26$) denotes patients with progressive or stable disease. The second and third columns show the responses to APD among those initially progressive (worsening) ($n = 17$), and those with initially stable scans ($n = 9$).

82

secutive scans: the nine remaining patients had stable scans. After treatment, scan appearances showed no further deterioration in five of these 17 patients, and one of the five showed objective regression. Of the remaining 12 patients with progressive scans four died, one withdrew before post-treatment assessment and seven had further progression. Of the nine patients with stable scans only one showed progression; the rest remained stable.

The effects of treatment on metabolic activity in bone are shown in Figures 2–6 inclusive. Fasting morning urinary hydroxyproline/creatinine ratios are plotted serially in Figures 2 and 3. Thirteen patients with high starting values are shown in Figure 2. Of these, nine had a significant fall at four weeks; this was sustained in seven at three months and in five at six months. Twelve of the remaining 13 who started treatment with normal values are shown in Figure 3. Five had sustained falls at six months; six showed a rise (in three cases

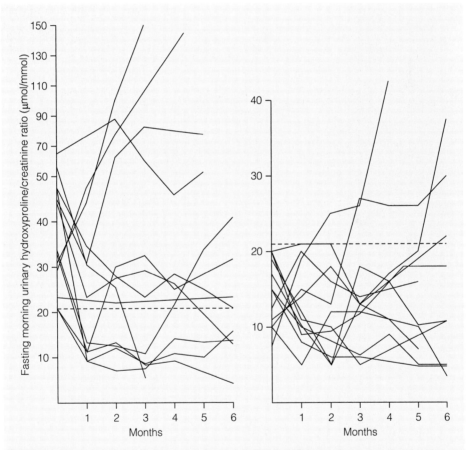

Fig. 2. The fasting morning urinary hydroxyproline/creatinine ratio in 13 patients with elevated baseline values. Compare with Figure 3, allowing for difference in scale.

Fig. 3. The fasting morning urinary hydroxyproline/creatinine ratio in 12 of the 13 patients with normal baseline values. Compare with Figure 2, allowing for difference in scale.

Table I. The Karnofsky performance score, a measure of mobility, where 100 indicates full mobility and 0 total immobility. The scores of patients receiving APD for metastatic cancer of the prostate were assessed before treatment, and at three and six months on treatment.

Score	Pretreatment ($n = 26$)	At three months ($n = 25$)	At six months ($n = 21$)
100	8	16	15
80–90	11	2	3
50–70	7	6	3
20–40	–	1	–
0–10	–	–	–

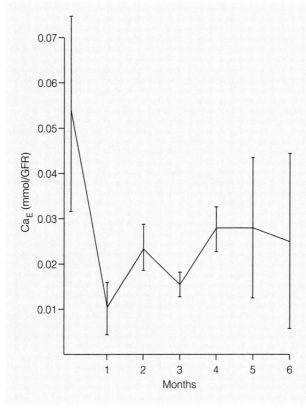

Fig. 4. The effect of APD on mean urinary calcium excretion (Ca_E) in 12 patients with progressive disease (bars indicate 95% confidence limits). $P < 0.0001$ at one month.

following a preliminary fall); one patient remained static. Data were incomplete for the final patient.

Figure 4 illustrates the effects of APD on mean urinary calcium excretion in the 12 patients with progressive disease. A highly significant fall is seen at one month ($P < 0.0001$), and this is sustained at six months. Similar effects are seen on mean serum osteocalcin values (Fig. 5), although the pattern of fall is

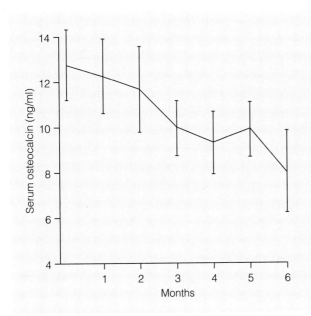

Fig. 5. The effect of APD on the mean serum osteocalcin values (bars indicate 95% confidence limits). $P<0.0001$ at three months.

slower. A significantly lower level is reached at three months ($P<0.0001$); thereafter levels continue to fall but not to a statistically significant degree.

The effect of APD on serum alkaline phosphatase in 18 patients with high serum levels at the onset of treatment is shown in Figure 6. Falling levels are seen in ten patients at four weeks, with continuing lower levels in seven patients at six months; one patient remained stable. Inexorable progression is seen in eight patients. Two patients died within six months, with alkaline phosphatase levels lowered but still high.

The effects of APD on bone histomorphometry were assessed by examining repeat tumour-free biopsies from 14 patients. Of the remaining 12 patients, five died or withdrew and therefore had no second biopsy; biopsy was unsuccessful in two patients, and the remainder had biopsies infiltrated by tumour. The results (Fig. 7) show that all patients had abnormally high peripheral bone resorption as judged by eroded surface. This fell significantly on treatment ($P<0.02$), and returned virtually to normal. A similar drop was seen in osteoid surface ($P<0.01$). Bone volume and mineralisation rate also showed significant falls over the six months ($P<0.01$ and 0.001 respectively).

The effects of APD on pain and mobility were assessed by the Karnofsky performance score, and by the analogue pain score (Table II). In the latter pain is graded from 0 (no pain) to 5 (intolerable pain). Before treatment eight patients were pain free, 11 had pain of grades 1 and 2 (mild to moderate), and seven had pain of grades 3 and 4 (severe to very severe). At three months, 25 patients were available for assessment: 15 were pain free, seven had pain of grades 1–2 (one of whom had undergone local palliative radiotherapy) and three remained on grades 3–4. At six months only 21 patients were available for assessment: 12 were pain free, nine had pain of grades 1–2, and none had pain of grades 3–4.

85

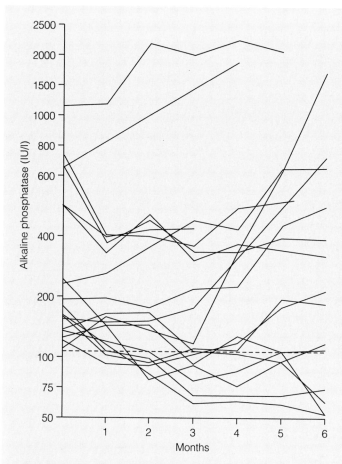

Fig. 6. The effect of APD on serum alkaline phosphatase in 18 patients with high serum levels at the start of APD therapy.

Mobility scores also improved. Scores of 100 were assigned to eight patients before treatment, to 16 after three months and to 15 at six months. Patients with improved scores came more frequently from among those with pretreatment scores in the 80–90 range, but some patients with pretreatment scores in the 60–70 range also benefited.

A number of patients needed fewer analgesics. Of six taking non-steroidal anti-inflammatory drugs, two reduced their dosage and four stopped altogether; of 11 using opiates, five increased their dosage, two remained on the same dose, three reduced their intake and one stopped analgesics completely.

The effect of APD on tumour markers was assessed by the serum prostatic acid phosphatase level, taken before and during treatment. Figure 8 shows serial values in 11 patients whose acid phosphatase was above the upper limit of normal at the start of treatment. Of these, six showed a fall. One of the six had undergone palliative radiotherapy two months prior to treatment. Levels continued to rise in the remaining five patients.

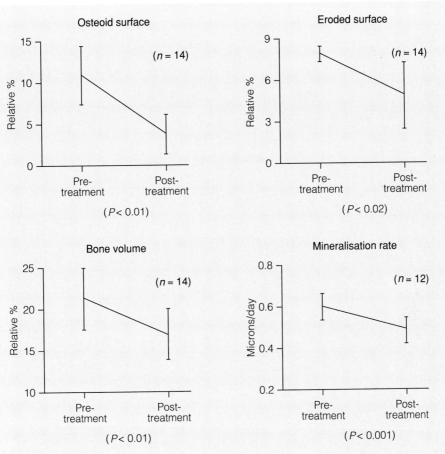

Fig. 7. Histomorphometric parameters (osteoid surface, eroded surface, bone volume and mineralisation rate) in repeat tumour-free biopsies from 14 patients, following treatment with APD.

Table II. The analogue pain score, in which pain is graded: 0 (no pain), 1 (mild), 2 (moderate), 3 (severe), 4 (very severe) or 5 (intolerable). The scores of patients receiving APD for metastatic cancer of the prostate were assessed before treatment, and at three and six months on treatment.

Score	Pretreatment ($n = 26$)	At three months ($n = 25$)	At six months ($n = 21$)
0	8	15	12
1–2	11	7	9
3–4	7	3	0
5	–	–	–

Conclusions

In some patients, APD diminishes abnormal metabolic activity in bone; it reduces tumour-free bone erosion, but also reduces bone volume and mineralisation rate. Progressive bone scans may stabilise and serum acid phosphatase levels fall in some patients. Subjectively, analogue pain scores fall and Karnofsky performance scores improve in a significant number and there may be a reduced need for analgesics.

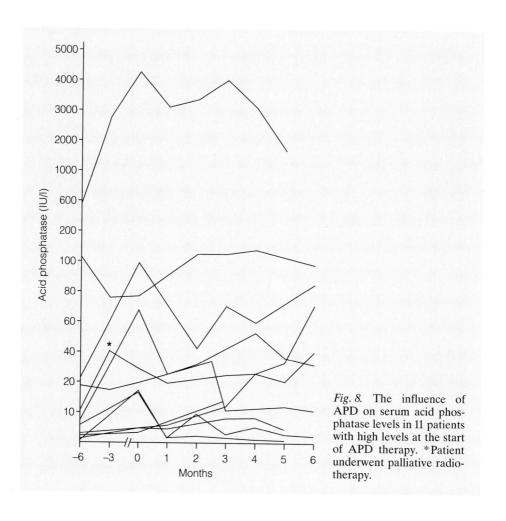

Fig. 8. The influence of APD on serum acid phosphatase levels in 11 patients with high levels at the start of APD therapy. *Patient underwent palliative radiotherapy.

References

JACOBS, S.C. (1983) Spread of prostate cancer to bone. *J. Urol. 21*, 337–344.
TATE, H.C., RAWLINSON, J.B. and FREEDMAN, L.S. (1979) Randomised comparative studies on the treatment of cancer in the United Kingdom: room for improvement? *Lancet ii*, 623–625.
WHITMORE, W.F. Jr (1956) Hormone therapy in prostate cancer. *Am. J. Med. 21*, 697–713.

Discussion

Dr A. EFREMIDIS (Athens): I do not understand the biological principle on which you based your study. APD inhibits osteoclast activity, but you have chosen a disease where osteoblastic activity is not necessarily related to increased osteoclastic activity.

CLARKE: It is a popular misconception that bone erosion does not occur in prostate cancer. In fact erosion in both tumour-free and tumour-affected bone is enormously elevated in patients with advanced prostatic disease – this has been proved biochemically and histomorphometrically.

EFREMIDIS: Then how do you know that response to APD is not due to a direct action on normal osteoblastic activity? You did not show the localised effects of APD, only generalised activity.

CLARKE: In the absence of definitive histological material – which we hope to present at further meetings – we have to rely on the global picture from serum markers and urine markers. We know what is happening in the peripheral skeleton from the histomorphometric data, but there are insufficient data to be sure what is happening histologically in the metastases. There is no doubt that, in a proportion of patients, the serum and urine markers do fall, suggesting a response within metastases.

Disodium pamidronate (APD) – a dose-seeking study in patients with breast and prostate cancer

A. Lipton[1], H. Harvey[1], E. Givant[1], N. Lipton[1], J. Lynch[1], J. Seaman[2],
C. Vandepol[2], D. Dellanno[2] and K. Zelenakas[2]

[1]Milton S. Hershey Medical Center, Hershey, Pennsylvania, USA, and
[2]Ciba-Geigy Corporation, Summit, New Jersey, USA

Summary

Disodium pamidronate (APD) is a new bisphosphonate and a potent inhibitor of osteoclastic bone resorption. In this dose-seeking trial, patients with symptomatic bone metastases from breast or prostate cancer were randomised to receive one of the following intravenous regimens – 30 mg every two weeks, 60 mg every two weeks, 60 mg every four weeks, or 90 mg every four weeks. To date, 12 breast and 13 prostate cancer patients have entered the trial. No haematological, biochemical or significant clinical toxicity has been observed. Of the ten breast cancer patients evaluable to date, all reported a decrease in pain; in some, analgesic requirements were lowered. Six of the 12 prostate cancer patients evaluable reported a decrease in pain. Our early impression is that pain relief is greater at the 60 and 90 mg doses. A consistent decline in serum and urine bone markers is seen in the patients with breast cancer. Objective evidence of bone healing has been observed in three patients with breast cancer and in one patient with prostatic cancer.

Introduction

Recent theory suggests that cancer cells produce mediators that result in the activation of osteoclasts. If this is true, and the malignant cell does not directly affect bone, alteration of osteoclast activity becomes the critical factor in determining whether the disease will progress in sites of metastatic involvement (Galasko and Bennett, 1976).

Disodium pamidronate (APD) is a new bisphosphonate that is a potent inhibitor of osteoclastic bone resorption, and does not inhibit bone formation. In three previous studies APD was used as palliative treatment for osteolytic metastases of breast cancer. Van Breukelen et al (1979) treated 14 patients with osteolytic bone disease – due to breast cancer or multiple myeloma – with an oral dose of APD of 60 µmol/kg/day. Biochemical markers for osteolytic activity, such as urinary hydroxyproline and serum calcium, decreased in most patients. In another study (van Holten-Verzantvoort et al, 1987), long-term oral treatment with APD 300 mg daily resulted in reduction of bone pain and fewer pathological fractures in patients with osteolytic metastases. In their study, Coleman et al (1988) treated 28 patients with advanced progressive symptomatic bone metastases with APD 30 mg intravenously, every two weeks for six months. Reduction in bone pain was frequently reported, and in four patients there was radiological evidence of bone healing.

In prostatic cancer, bone metastases are usually osteoblastic, rather than the mixed lytic-blastic lesions seen in breast cancer. To date, there is little experience of treating the bone metastases of prostatic cancer with APD (CLARKE and GEORGE, 1990).

The aims of the present study were as follows:
- to confirm that APD can bring about pain relief in patients with symptomatic bone metastases from breast and prostatic cancer,
- to determine the optimal intravenous dose of APD, and
- to see if objective response could be achieved in bone metastases from breast and prostatic cancer.

Patient population

All patients had bone metastases from breast or prostatic cancer that had failed to respond to at least one previous systemic treatment. Entry criteria were:
- aged 18 years or over
- an estimated life expectancy of at least three months
- an overall bone pain score of at least 4 (see Table I and below)
- no radiation therapy in the two weeks preceding or at any time during the trial
- satisfactory blood picture (haematocrit $>30\%$, WBC $>3.5 \times 10^9/l$, platelets $>100 \times 10^9/l$, serum creatinine <200 μmol/l, bilirubin <25 μmol/l), and
- no clinically significant changes on the electrocardiogram.

Cancer chemotherapy, corticosteroids and hormonal therapy were not permitted in the two weeks preceding the study or during the trial period, unless the patient had been on continuous or cyclical treatment with no change in the 60 days prior to beginning APD.

Drug schedules

Following informed consent, patients were randomised to one of four treatment regimens:
- Treatment A: 30 mg APD intravenously once every two weeks
- Treatment B: 60 mg APD intravenously once every two weeks
- Treatment C: 60 mg APD intravenously once every four weeks
- Treatment D: 90 mg APD intravenously once every four weeks.

Treatments A, B and C were infused over four hours, treatment D over six hours.

Patient evaluation

Patients were evaluated by history and physical examination every 14 days. Each patient kept a daily diary of symptoms and medication. Pain was assessed on visual analogue scales for severity and frequency and recorded as an overall pain score, representing their product (Table I). Use of analgesics was as-

Table I. Assessment of the pain score at the treatment site.

Pain score = Pain severity × Pain frequency

– where severity is rated:
  0 = None
  1 = Mild
  2 = Moderate
  3 = Severe

and

– where frequency is rated:
  0 = No pain
  1 = Occasional (less than daily)
  2 = Intermittent (at least once a day)
  3 = Constant (most of the time)

---

sessed by a narcotic score (recorded as the product of the type of drug used and the frequency of use) (Table II). Performance status was recorded according to the Karnofsky and the Eastern Cooperative Oncology Group criteria. Biochemical tests were performed every two weeks, and included a complete blood count with differential, platelet count, urinalysis, blood glucose, screening tests for liver and renal function (automated SMAC), calcium, phosphorus, magnesium, alkaline phosphatase (total and bone isozyme), serum osteocalcin, prostate-specific antigen, acid phosphatase, and two-hour fasting urine for calcium/creatinine and hydroxyproline/creatinine ratios. Bone scan and bone survey were used as objective evidence of response, and were performed at three-month intervals.

Table II. Assessment of the narcotic score.

Narcotic Score = Medication type × Medication frequency

– where drug type is graded:
  0 = None
  1 = Analgesic (e.g. aspirin with any OTC component, propoxephene, etc.)
  2 = Mild narcotic (e.g. 30 mg codeine, oxycodone, meperidine, etc.)
  3 = Strong narcotic (e.g. 60 mg or more of codeine, morphine, hydromorphone, etc.)

and

– where frequency is graded:
  0 = None
  1 = Less than daily
  2 = Once per day
  3 = More than once per day

Results in breast cancer

Twelve patients with symptomatic bone metastases from breast cancer have so far entered the trial. One patient had to be withdrawn from the trial because a nerve block had to be performed in the only painful area, while another has so far received only a single dose of APD. There are thus ten patients for evaluation.

Subjective response to APD was reported by all ten patients, and was confirmed by a fall in pain score from an initial mean value of 5.8 to a mean value of 3.8 ($P = 0.005$) after 12 weeks on the protocol (Fig. 1). Similarly, the mean baseline visual analogue score was 6.5, but this dropped to 3.5 ($P < 0.01$) after three months. The mean narcotic score also dropped significantly ($P = 0.04$) from a mean value of 6.2 to 5.2 after three months (Fig. 2). Patients frequently reported a decrease in bone pain 1–3 days after receiving APD, but symptoms would often worsen in the fourth week in those patients receiving APD every four weeks.

No change was observed in the serum calcium during the initial three-month treatment period (Fig. 3); however, there were falls in the bone alkaline phosphatase and in the urinary calcium/creatinine and hydroxyproline/creatinine ratios ($P = 0.07$, 0.27 and 0.03 respectively). At the moment the number of patients in this trial is too small to permit any deduction about the optimal APD dose.

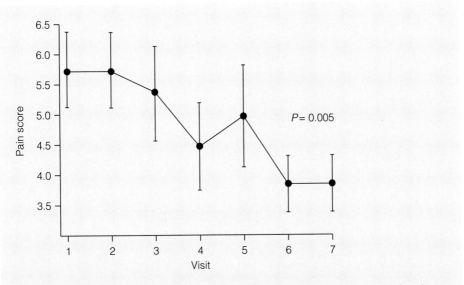

Fig. 1. Mean pain score ($\pm$ standard error) in patients with breast cancer metastatic to bone during the first three months of treatment with APD (visit 1 = before starting APD treatment; each subsequent visit at two weekly intervals).

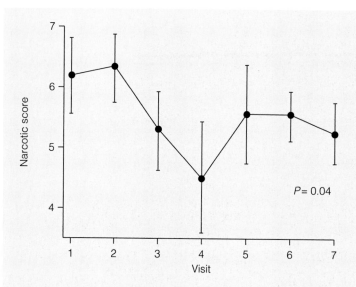

Fig. 2. Mean narcotic score (± standard error) in patients with breast cancer metastatic to bone during the first three months of treatment with APD. Compare with Figure 1.

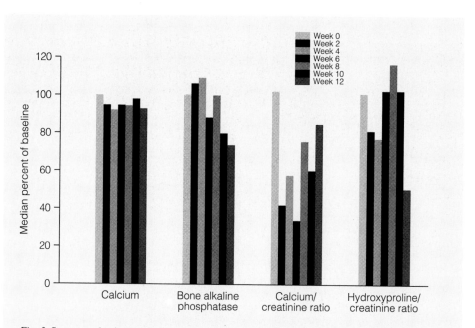

Fig. 3. Serum and urinary biochemical markers in patients with breast cancer metastatic to bone during the first three months of treatment with APD.

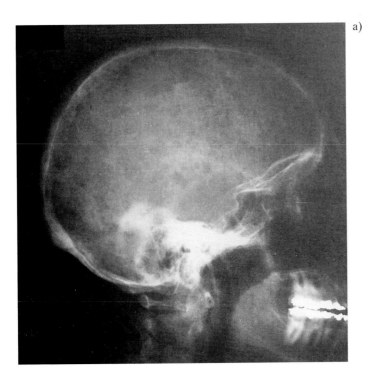

a)

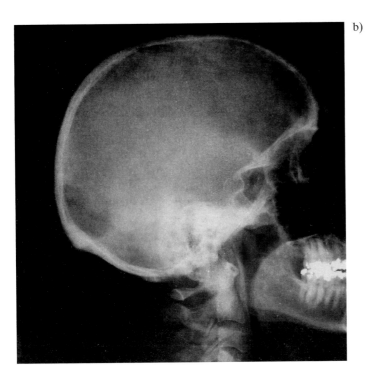

b)

Fig. 4. New sclerotic areas in skull consistent with bone healing in a patient with metastatic breast carcinoma (a) prior to treatment, and (b) after three months' treatment with APD.

Three patients showed objective evidence of bone healing. In one, osteoblastic skull metastases disappeared; in the other two, sclerotic areas appeared in sites of previous osteolytic disease (Figs 4 and 5). It is of interest that all three had received treatment D (90 mg APD every four weeks). To date, one patient among the ten has shown progression of bone disease.

Results in prostatic cancer

Thirteen patients with symptomatic bone metastases from prostate cancer received treatment with APD. One patient was randomised to treatment A, but then decided that he did not wish to participate in the trial, thus leaving 12 patients for evaluation.

Subjective response to APD was reported by six patients, and was confirmed by a fall in pain score from an initial mean value of 5.9 to a mean value of 4.5 ($P = 0.06$) after 12 weeks on the protocol (Fig. 6). Similarly, the mean baseline visual analogue score was 4.7, but this dropped to a low of 2.5, and to 4.2 ($P = 0.01$) after three months. The mean narcotic score did not change significantly in patients with prostatic cancer ($P = 0.9$).

As in the patients with breast cancer, no change was observed in the serum calcium during the initial three-month treatment period (Fig. 7); acid phosphatase and prostate-specific antigen levels were also unchanged. Slight falls in both the urinary calcium/creatinine and hydroxyproline/creatinine ratios were also noted, but bone alkaline phosphatase remained unchanged (Fig. 7).

One patient showed objective evidence of bone healing (Fig. 8), and so far has received 30 mg APD every two weeks for more than eight months. While receiving APD, two patients showed disease progression in bone, while four others suffered progression of their prostatic cancer in sites other than bone.

Toxicity

No haematological or biochemical changes have been observed in the 24 patients treated with APD. Five had a 'flu-like' syndrome that usually occurred during the first three treatments and then abated: symptoms consisted of mild fever, chills and malaise occurring within 24–72 hours of receiving APD and lasting 12–24 hours.

Two patients with prostatic cancer developed clinical signs of spinal cord compression – this was not observed in the breast cancer patients. We suggest that when APD is being considered for patients with spinal metastases, magnetic resonance imaging of the spine and/or a myelogram be performed prior to treatment.

Two patients – one from each group – died from a rapidly progressive interstitial pneumonic process, probably due to progressive lymphangitic disease.

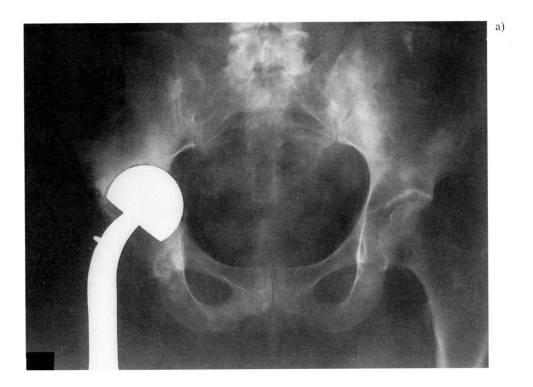

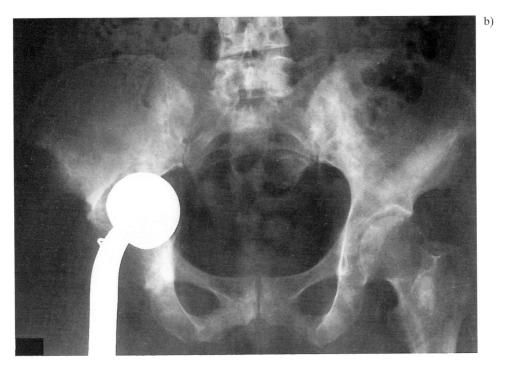

Fig. 5. New sclerotic areas consistent with bone healing in a patient with metastatic breast carcinoma (a) prior to treatment, and (b) after three months' treatment with APD.

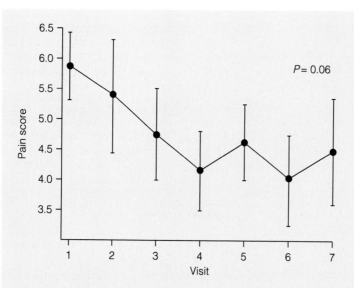

Fig. 6. Mean pain score (± standard error) in patients with prostate cancer metastatic to bone during the first three months of treatment with APD.

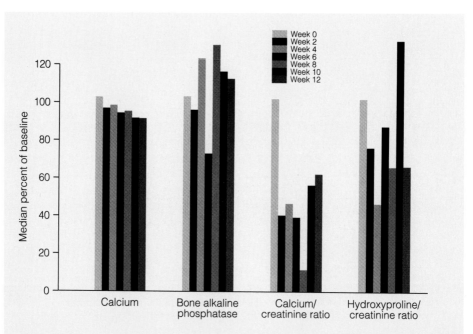

Fig. 7. Serum and urinary biochemical markers in patients with prostate cancer metastatic to bone during the first three months of treatment with APD.

Discussion and conclusions

It is a new concept to protect a site in the body from progression of cancer rather than attempting to kill the cancer cells directly. Bisphosphonates such as APD are potent inhibitors of osteoclastic bone resorption and are not known to have any direct antitumour effects.

This report is an early analysis of an ongoing clinical trial employing the new bisphosphonate disodium pamidronate (APD) in patients with bone metastases from breast and prostatic cancer. All patients entering this study had progressive, painful bone disease after at least one previous systemic treatment. Despite the fact that this trial is still in the early stages, several conclusions emerge:

- APD is well tolerated.
- Treatment with APD can achieve a reduction in bone pain in both groups of patients.
- A consistent decline in serum and urine bone markers is seen in breast cancer patients.
- Objective evidence of bone healing has been observed in both groups.

It is our early impression that breast cancer patients respond more frequently and for longer than do patients with metastatic prostate cancer; this may suggest differences in the mechanism of bone metastases in the two diseases.

a)   b)

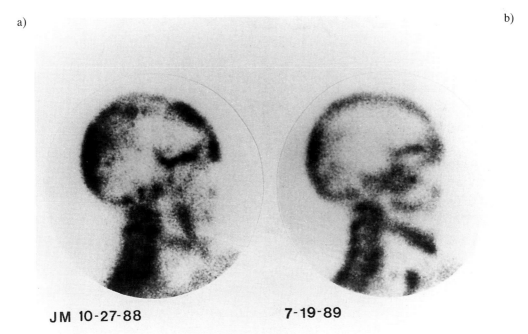

JM 10-27-88   7-19-89

Fig. 8. Bone scans showing disappearance of hot spots, consistent with bone healing in a patient with metastatic carcinoma of the prostate treated with APD (a) before treatment, and (b) after three months' treatment with APD.

Bone metastases from breast cancer are usually both lytic and blastic, while those from prostate cancer are usually wholly blastic in nature. Nevertheless, there is no doubt that certain patients with prostate cancer show both subjective and objective response to APD therapy. It is interesting that the one objective response occurred in a patient who had received APD at low dose for a period of eight months.

Further work is needed to determine the optimal dose and schedule for APD. Several early studies used oral APD but, in view of the variable absorption that occurs with an oral agent, we recommend intravenous administration until more is known about the drug. The three objective responses in breast cancer were all in patients treated with 90 mg APD every four weeks. This is important, as most European studies have used APD in doses of 45 mg or less. Symptomatic relief lasts approximately three weeks in patients receiving APD at monthly intervals, suggesting that a four-weekly schedule may be too long. In summary, APD is a well tolerated therapy that can be of great subjective and objective benefit to certain patients with bone metastases from breast or prostate cancer.

Acknowledgement

The authors wish to thank Mrs Michelle Moore for help in preparing the manuscript.

References

CLARKE, N.W., McCLURE, J. and GEORGE, N.J.R. (1990) Subjective and metabolic effects of aminohydroxypropylidine bisphosphonate (APD) in patients with advanced cancer of the prostate: a preliminary report. In: *The Management of Bone Metastases and Hypercalcaemia by Osteoclast Inhibition,* R.D. Rubens (Ed.), pp. 81–89. Hogrefe and Huber, Toronto/Lewiston NY/Bern/Göttingen/Stuttgart.

COLEMAN, R.E., WOLL, P. and RUBENS, R.D. (1988) Bisphosphonate treatment of bone metastases from breast cancer. Abstract 789. *Am. Assoc. Cancer Res. 29,* 199.

GALASKO, C.S.B. and BENNETT, A. (1976) Mechanism of bone destruction in the development of skeletal metastases. *Nature 263,* 507–508.

VAN BREUKELEN, F.J.M., BIJVOET, O.L.M. and VAN OOSTEROM, A.T. (1979) Inhibition of osteolytic bone lesions by 3-amino-1-hydroxypropylidene-1,1-bisphosphonate (APD). *Lancet i,* 803–805.

VAN HOLTEN-VERZANTVOORT, A.T., BIJVOET, O.L.M., CLETON, F.J. et al (1987) Reduced morbidity from skeletal metastases in breast cancer patients during long-term bisphosphonate (APD) treatment. *Lancet ii,* 983–985.

A randomised trial of aminoglutethimide and hydrocortisone with and without disodium pamidronate (APD) in patients with advanced breast cancer

A. L. Harris[1], J. Carmichael[1], K. Tonkin[1], B. M. J. Cantwell[2], M. Millward[2] and K. Mannix[2]

[1]Imperial Cancer Research Fund Clinical Oncology Unit, Churchill Hospital, Headington, Oxford, UK, and [2]Clinical Oncology Unit, Newcastle General Hospital, Newcastle upon Tyne, UK

Summary

Short-duration APD infusions were assessed at two dose levels in patients with hypercalcaemia of malignancy. In the first study, 16 patients were given 30 mg APD intravenously over two hours; ten also received intravenous hydration. Calcium levels decreased significantly in all patients – in 15 to 2.77 mmol/l or less; mild hypocalcaemia occurred in two patients. Hypercalcaemia was controlled for a median of 13 days (range 10–69 days).

In a subsequent series of 25 patients (study 2), 45 mg APD was infused over three hours; all patients were hydrated. Twenty-four responded, and in 18 calcium levels fell to normal (<2.75 mmol/l). Five developed hypocalcaemia. Hypercalcaemia was controlled for a median of 19 days (range 11–62 days).

In the third study, based on the above data, 55 postmenopausal patients (all with bone secondaries from breast cancer) were randomised into two groups. All received low-dose aminoglutethimide (125 mg bd) and hydrocortisone (20 mg bd) as standard hormone therapy; in addition, one group received a three-weekly infusion of APD 30 mg. At 12 weeks, in the control group six patients showed objective response and three had stable disease. In the APD-treated group five showed objective response and four had stable disease. In each group 16 patients showed progressive disease by 12 weeks. Subsequent complications of bone metastases were not significantly different in the two groups. Among those treated with APD, actuarial survival at 1.5 years was 30%, compared with 10% without APD; progression-free survival at one year was zero without APD, 20% with APD.

Introduction

Bone is one of the commonest sites of metastasis in breast cancer; a recent review (Coleman and Rubens, 1987a) showed that bone metastases occurred in 69% of 587 patients dying from breast cancer, pathological fractures in 16% and spinal cord compression in 3%. Patients with bone metastases live longer than those with visceral metastases, and median survival times of 16–24 months have been reported (Clark et al, 1987; Romin and Donegan, 1987; Van de Velde et al, 1986). Hypercalcaemia occurs in 17% of these patients. Bone metastases are thus a major problem in breast cancer management.

Conventional treatment comprises local radiotherapy and systemic hormone therapy or chemotherapy. Recently, the ability of bisphosphonates to control hypercalcaemia of malignancy has been investigated (SLEEBOOM et al, 1983; RALSTON et al, 1985; COLEMAN and RUBENS, 1987b; BODY et al, 1987). Bisphosphonates have a P-C-P structure and bind with very high affinity to bone mineral matrix (POWELL and DEMARK, 1985). They can alter the surface charge on hydroxyapatite crystals (ROBERTSON et al, 1972), and inhibit bone resorption. They also appear to exert a direct effect on osteoclasts (BOONEKAMP et al, 1987), with nuclear aberrations and lysosomal abnormalities occurring after bisphosphonate therapy (PLASMANS et al, 1980). Other actions include prevention of osteoclast attachment to the bone matrix (FLEISCH, 1983), and inhibition of osteoclast differentiation and recruitment (BOONEKAMP et al, 1986).

The bisphosphonate APD (3-amino-1-hydroxypropylidene-1,1-bisphosphonate) has been used in a range of different schedules to treat hypercalcaemia. It was initially used at a dose of 15 mg daily for several days (SLEEBOOM et al, 1983). In order to use APD for outpatients it was necessary to develop a single-dose schedule that could be repeated on a regular basis. On the assumption that the mechanisms relating to hypercalcaemia in breast cancer were similar to those relating to progressive local destruction of bone, we decided to evaluate the effects of two single-dose schedules of intravenous APD in the control of hypercalcaemia, the development of hypocalcaemia, and duration of action (studies 1 and 2). Based on these data, we then used APD 30 mg once every three weeks in a randomised study with or without low-dose aminoglutethimide plus hydrocortisone in advanced breast cancer (study 3).

Patients and methods

In the first study, 16 patients were treated with intravenous APD 30 mg in 500 ml normal saline, infused over two hours. Ten of them received intravenous hydration with three litres of normal saline over 24 hours, starting at the same time as the APD infusion; six received APD alone. In the second study, 25 patients were treated with intravenous APD 45 mg in 750 ml normal saline, infused over three hours. All received hydration simultaneously with the APD infusion. The pretreatment characteristics of both groups of patients are shown in Table I, which includes patients with lung and other cancers.

In the third study, 55 postmenopausal patients with breast cancer and metastatic bone disease were randomised to receive low-dose aminoglutethimide 125 mg bd and hydrocortisone 20 mg bd, with or without APD. Those randomised to receive APD were given 30 mg in 500 ml normal saline over two hours every three weeks. A total of 12 doses were given on an outpatient basis (as in study 1). Disease was assessed by X-ray appearances, bone scans, calcium excretion, CEA (carcinoembryonic antigen), osteocalcin, and alkaline phosphatase. Initial assessment was made at three months, and UICC criteria (HAYWARD et al, 1977) were used throughout.

Plasma calcium levels were estimated using a Technicon Autoanalyser and were corrected for the albumin concentration measured simultaneously, according to the formula: Corrected calcium = actual calcium ± 0.02 for each

Table I. Characteristics of patients in studies 1 and 2, who received APD alone in the treatment of hypercalcaemia.

	APD dose (mg)	n	M/F	Breast cancer	Lung or other squamous cancer	Cancer in other sites	Failure of previous treatment	Severe hypercalcae-mia (>3.5 mmol)
Study 1	30	16	11/5	5	9	2	2	5
Study 2	45	25	15/10	7	14	4	16	15

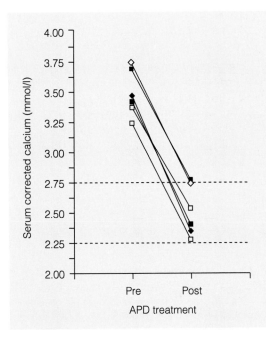

Fig. 1. Decrease in serum corrected calcium in the six patients in study 1 treated with APD but without hydration.

gram of albumin above or below 40 g/l (EDITORIAL, 1977). Our normal range is 2.25–2.75 mmol/l.

Results

Study 1. The serum calcium decreased in all patients. Normocalcaemia was achieved in 12 out of 16 (75%), and in three of the four remaining patients it fell below 2.8 mmol/l. Median duration of response was 13 days (range 10–69 days). In the six patients treated with APD alone (without hydration), the elevated pretreatment calcium levels fell to normal in each case (Fig. 1). The

103

Table II. Response of patients in studies 1 and 2 to the two different doses of APD (30 mg and 45 mg respectively).

	APD dose (mg)	n	Serum calcium: Normalised (2.25–2.75 mmol/l)	Hypo (<2.25 mmol/l)	Hyper (2.75–3.10 mmol/l)	Resis-tant	Severe hypercalcaemia (>3.5 mmol/l) Normalised	Fall
							(n = 4)	
Study 1	30	16	10	2 (2.08/2.18)	4	0	1	2
							(n = 15)	
Study 2	45	25	13	5 (>1.99)	6	1	9	4

	Previous treatment failure Normalised	Fall	Median time to fall in days (range)	Median duration of response in days (range)
	(n = 2)			
Study 1	1	1	4 (1–9)	13 (10–69)
	(n = 16)			
Study 2	11	5	6 (2–10)	19 (11–62)

time to achieve normocalcaemia ranged from one to nine days (median five days) (CANTWELL and HARRIS, 1987).

Study 2. In this consecutive series more serious hypercalcaemia was present; 15 out of 25 patients had a serum calcium above 3.5 mmol/l, compared to only four out of 16 in the previous study. Also, more patients had previously failed to respond to other antihypercalcaemic therapy, including frusemide, calcitonin, mithramycin and glucocorticoids: 16 out of 25, compared to only two out of 16 in study 1 (Table I). However, normocalcaemia was achieved in 13 and hypocalcaemia in five. Median duration of control was longer in this series (Table II) but, while none of the lung cancer patients had their hypercalcaemia controlled for more than 18 days, four out of seven patients with breast cancer were controlled for longer (MANNIX et al, 1989).

Study 3. Based on previous toxicity and therapeutic studies with APD, we believed that 30 mg APD every three weeks would be an effective dose, with little risk of hypocalcaemia. Pretreatment characteristics of the patients in this study are shown in Table III; most had been extensively pretreated with at least one hormone therapy, and many had also received chemotherapy and radiotherapy for bone secondaries. Response to previous hormone therapy is an important prognostic indicator for response to further courses of hormone therapy; the two arms of the trial were well balanced in this regard (Table IV), and also with regard to other visceral sites of disease (Table III).

Table III. Pretreatment characteristics of patients in study 3, divided into two groups: those receiving only aminoglutethimide and hydrocortisone (AG/HC), and those receiving APD in addition (AG/HC/APD).

	AG/HC (n = 28)	AG/HC/APD (n = 27)
Age (range)	59 years (36–85)	53 years (32–72)
Weight in kg (range)	61 (48–80)	65 (40–94)
Sites of disease		
– Bone alone	9	8
– Bone + local spread	8	10
– Bone + distant metastases	11	9
Sites of distant metastases		
– Lung	6	2
– Liver	5	7
– Pleura	2	1
– Other (intra-abdominal, mediastinal)	3	1
Previous hormone therapy		
– Tamoxifen	24	22
– Oophorectomy	4	5
– Others (MPA, LHRH agonist, anandron)	4	5
Previous chemotherapy		
– Mitozantrone, adriamycin, MMC/VCR, Adr/Ifos, CMF	8	7
No previous therapy	2	2
Disease-free interval in months (range)	26 (0–149)	21 (0–93)
Time from last menstrual period (years)	12	8

Table IV. Outcome of previous hormone and chemotherapy among patients in study 3, divided into two groups: those receiving only aminoglutethimide and hydrocortisone (AG/HC), and those receiving APD in addition (AG/HC/APD).

	AG/HC (n = 28)	AG/HC/APD (n = 27)
Positive response to hormones*	9	11
Positive response to chemotherapy*	3	5
No response to hormones	0	4
No response to chemotherapy	1	0
Unknown/unassessable	11	8

* Including stable disease for more than three months

105

At 12 weeks there were nine responders, including stable disease, in both arms of the trial. In four patients it was too early to assess response. Similarly, 16 patients in each group had progressed by 12 weeks (Table V). At 24 weeks there were also no significant differences in response (Table VI).

Subsequent complications of bone metastases (analysed to 24. 7. 89) show no significant differences between the two groups (Table VII). However, there have been 13 pathological events in the 27 patients receiving APD, compared with 19 in the 28 patients not receiving it.

Peto log rank analysis shows no significant differences in overall survival or in progression-free survival in the two groups. However, at one year all patients not receiving APD had progressed, whereas 20% of those on APD remained in remission. Actuarial survival at 1.5 years was only 10% in those not receiving APD compared to 30% in those on APD (Figs 2 and 3). However, the numbers of patients involved are small.

Table V. Outcome at 12 weeks among patients in study 3, divided into two groups: those receiving only aminoglutethimide and hydrocortisone (AG/HC), and those receiving APD in addition (AG/HC/APD).

	AG/HC ($n = 28$)	AG/HC/APD ($n = 27$)
Early progression (before 12 weeks)	10	6
Progressive disease	6	10
Stable disease	3	4
Positive response	6	5
Too early to assess	2	2
Not assessable	1	0

Table VI. Outcome at 24 weeks among patients in study 3, divided into two groups: those receiving only aminoglutethimide and hydrocortisone (AG/HC), and those receiving APD in addition (AG/HC/APD).

	AG/HC ($n = 28$)	AG/HC/APD ($n = 27$)
Early progression (before 12 weeks)	10	6
Progressive disease	7	10
Stable disease	1	2
Positive response	6	5
Too early to assess	3	4
Not assessable	1	0

Table VII. Subsequent complications among patients in study 3, divided into two groups: those receiving only aminoglutethimide and hydrocortisone (AG/HC), and those receiving APD in addition (AG/HC/APD).

	AG/HC ($n = 28$)	AG/HC/APD ($n = 27$)
Pathological fracture	3	3
Spinal cord compression	2	0
Radiotherapy to bone metastases	12	10
Hypercalcaemia of malignancy	2	0

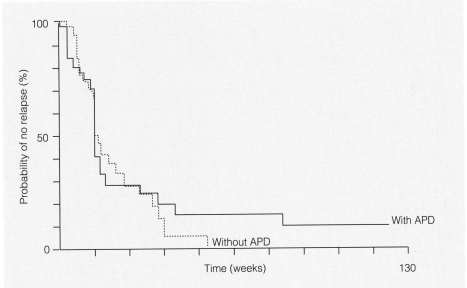

Fig. 2. Percentage probability of not suffering a relapse among patients in study 3, divided into two groups: those receiving APD and those not receiving it.

Discussion of study 3

This study confirmed our earlier data, indicating that low-dose aminoglutethimide and hydrocortisone is a well tolerated endocrine therapy with activity in advanced breast cancer (HARRIS et al, 1989). Our initial assessment shows no statistically significant evidence of improved response by the addition of APD, either in reducing the complications of bone metastasis or in overall survival. There are several possible reasons for this. Many patients had been heavily pretreated with hormone therapy, and the overall response rate would therefore be lower. Moreover, confidence intervals on the data currently available are wide.

107

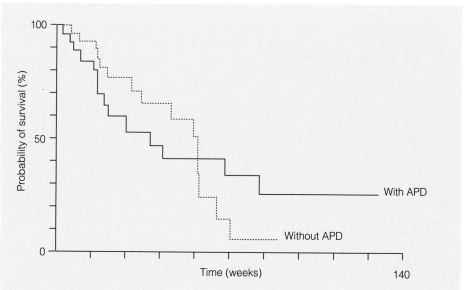

Fig. 3. Percentage probability of survival among patients in study 3, divided into two groups: those receiving APD and those not receiving it.

Two previous studies using APD 30 mg alone for the treatment of osteolytic bone secondaries in breast cancer have shown objective responses. COLEMAN et al (1988) had four objective responses in 28 patients, MORTON et al (1988b) had four in 16 patients: both had a further subgroup of patients with stable disease for at least three months. These studies used APD every two weeks, in contrast to our three-weekly schedule. However, in an earlier study, MORTON et al (1988a) showed that 30 mg APD given every three weeks could control hypercalcaemia, confirming our earlier report (CANTWELL and HARRIS, 1987). Although it is possible that our schedule is less effective, it is more likely that the two modalities of treatment – APD and hormone therapy – are interacting in the same sensitive group of patients. Hence, there is no marked improvement in response *rate* although one might expect an improved *duration* of response, as seems to be occurring in our present study.

Two randomised studies using daily *oral* bisphosphonates have been reported (ELOMAA et al, 1983 and 1985). In the first, there was a reduction both in hypercalcaemia and in the number of new metastases in patients on bisphosphonate after one year's therapy. During the second year of follow-up, there was a much lower incidence of hypercalcaemia and pathological fracture in the bisphosphonate group, and an improved incidence of survival. However, the study suffered from a lack of detailed comparison of prognostic factors and concomitant therapies, and there was no statistical analysis.

In the second, larger study (VAN HOLTEN-VERZANTVOORT et al, 1987) oral APD was added to a variety of systemic therapies, resulting in a significant reduction in hypercalcaemia, bone pain, pathological fracture, and the need for radiotherapy. There was, however, no difference in survival time, and the benefits of APD did not emerge until after six months of therapy. Most of our patients have not yet been followed up for six months.

In conclusion, our study shows the feasibility of combining APD with aminoglutethimide and hydrocortisone, and is the first study of its use in patients on uniform endocrine management. Early analysis shows more events relating to bone secondaries in the control group, and more long-term survivors in the treated group. These results are not as yet statistically significant, and it is planned to double the study size. Ultimately, the best way to combine bisphosphonates with hormone therapy is likely to be continuous daily oral administration.

Acknowledgement

We thank Ciba-Geigy for supplying disodium pamidronate (APD) and for funding specialist chemotherapy nurses.

References

BODY, J.-J., POT, M., BORKOWSKI, A. et al (1987) Dose/response study of aminohydroxypropylidine bisphosphonate in tumor-associated hypercalcemia. *Am. J. Med. 82*, 957–963.

BOONEKAMP, P. M., VAN DER WEE-PALS, L. J. A., VAN WIJK-VAN LENNEP, M. M. L. et al (1986) Two modes of action of bisphosphonates on osteolytic resorption of mineralized bone matrix. *Bone Min. 1*, 27–40.

BOONEKAMP, P. M., LÖWICK, G. W. G. M., VAN DER WEE-PALS, L. J. A. et al (1987) Enhancement of the inhibitory action of APD on the transformation of osteoclast precursors into resorbing cells after demethylation of the amino group. *Bone Min. 2*, 29–42.

CANTWELL, B. M. J. and HARRIS, A. L. (1987) Effect of single high dose infusions of aminohydroxyprophylidine bisphosphonate on hypercalcaemia caused by cancer. *Br. Med. J. 294*, 467–469.

CLARK, G. M., SLEDGE, G. W., OSBORNE, K. et al (1987) Survival from first recurrence: Relative importance of prognostic factors in 1,015 breast cancer patients. *J. Clin. Oncol. 5*, 55–61.

COLEMAN, R. E. and RUBENS, R. D. (1987a) The clinical course of bone metastases. *Br. J. Cancer 13*, 89–94.

COLEMAN, R. E. and RUBENS, R. D. (1987b) Treatment of hypercalcaemia secondary to advanced breast cancer with 3-amino-1,1-hydroxypropylidene bisphosphonate (APD) *Br. J. Cancer 56*, 465–469.

COLEMAN, R. E., WOLL, P. J., MILES, M. et al (1988) Treatment of bone metastases from breast cancer with 3-amino-1-hydroxypropylidene-1,1-bisphosphonate (APD). *Br. J. Cancer 58*, 621–625.

EDITORIAL (1977) Correcting the calcium. *Br. Med. J. 1*, 598.

ELOMAA, I., BLOMQVIST, C., GROHN, P. et al (1983) Long-term controlled trial with diphosphonate in patients with osteolytic bone metastases. *Lancet i*, 146–149.

ELOMAA, I., BLOMQVIST, C. and PORKKA, L. (1985) Diphosphonates for osteolytic bone metastases. *Lancet i*, 1155–1156.

FLEISCH, H. (1983) Bisphosphonates: Mechanisms of action and clinical applications. In: *Bone and Mineral Research*, Annual 1, W. A. Peck (Ed.), pp. 319–357. Excerpta Medica, Amsterdam.

HARRIS, A. L., CANTWELL, B. M. J., CARMICHAEL, J. et al (1989) Phase II study of low dose aminoglutethimide 250 mg/day plus hydrocortisone in advanced postmenopausal breast cancer. *Eur. J. Cancer Clin. Oncol. 25*, 1105–1111.

HAYWARD, J. L., CARBONE, P. P., HEUSON, J.-C. et al (1977) Assessment of response to therapy in advanced breast cancer. *Eur. J. Cancer 13*, 89–94.

MANNIX, K. A., CARMICHAEL, J., HARRIS, A. L. et al (1989) Single high-dose (45 mg) infusions of aminohydroxypropylidene diphosphonate for severe malignant hypercalcemia. *Cancer 64,* 1358–1361.

MORTON, A. R., CANTRILL, J. A., CRAIG, A. E. et al (1988a) Single dose versus daily intravenous aminohydroxyprophylidine biphosphonate (APD) for the hypercalcaemia of malignancy. *Br. Med. J. 296,* 811–814.

MORTON, A. R., CANTRILL, J. A., PILAI, G. V. et al (1988b) Sclerosis of lytic bone metastases after aminohydroxypropylidine bisphosphonate (APD) in patients with breast carcinoma. *Br. Med. J. 297,* 772–773.

PLASMANS, C. M. T., JAP, P. H. K., KUIJPERS, W. et al (1980) Influence of a diphosphonate on the cellular aspects of young bone tissue. *Calcif. Tissue Int. 32,* 247.

POWELL, J. H. and DEMARK, B. R. (1985) Clinical pharmacokinetics of diphosphonates. In: *Bone Resorption Metastasis and Diphosphonates,* S. Garratini (Ed.), pp. 41–49. Raven Press, New York.

RALSTON, S. H., GARDNER, M. D., DRYBURGH, F. J. et al (1985) Comparison of amino-hydroxypropylidine diphosphonate, mithramycin and corticosteroid/calcitonin in treatment of cancer-associated hypercalcaemia. *Lancet ii,* 906–910.

ROBERTSON, W. G., MORGAN, D. B., FLEISCH, H. et al (1972) The effects of diphosphonates on the exchangeable and non-exchangeable calcium and phosphate of hydroxyapatite. *Biochim. Biophys. Acta 261,* 517.

ROMIN, R. and DONEGAN, W. L. (1987) Screening for recurrent breast cancer – its effectiveness and prognostic value. *J. Clin. Oncol. 5,* 62–67.

SLEEBOOM, H. P., BIJVOET, O. L. M., VAN OOSTEROM, A. T. et al (1983) Comparison of intravenous (3-amino-1-hydroxypropylidene)-1,1-bisphosphonate and volume repletion in tumour-induced hypercalcaemia. *Lancet ii,* 239–243.

VAN DE VELDE, C. J. H., GALLAGER, H. S. and GIACCO, G. G. (1986) Prognosis in node-negative breast cancer. *Breast Cancer Res. Treat. 8,* 189.

VAN HOLTEN-VERZANTVOORT, A. T., BIJVOET, O. L. M., HERMANS, J. et al (1987) Reduced morbidity from skeletal metastases in breast cancer patients during long-term bisphosphonate (APD) treatment. *Lancet ii,* 983–985.

110

Are all anticancer effects of pamidronate (APD) and related compounds bone-mediated?

F. Wingen, T. Klenner and D. Schmähl
Institute of Toxicology and Chemotherapy, German Cancer Research
Centre, Heidelberg, Federal Republic of Germany

Summary

Until recently, pamidronate (APD) was thought to have no antitumour activity, and to act against bone metastases only by inhibiting the activity of osteoclasts or precursor cells. Now, using a slow-growing autochthonous mammary carcinoma in rats induced by methylnitrosourea, APD has been shown to have a significant antineoplastic action on the primary tumour.

We have investigated the antitumour activity of APD and other compounds, alone or in combination, in this model. APD combined with melphalan strongly inhibited the development of new tumours, whereas APD combined with tamoxifen was not effective. APD may exert its anticancer activity, alone or in combination with melphalan, by inhibiting malignant transformation of the methylnitrosourea-induced adenomas.

Introduction

3-amino-1-hydroxypropylidene-1,1-bisphosphonic acid (pamidronate, APD) has been found to be a potent inhibitor of osteoclasts, and this has led to its use in the treatment and prevention of hypercalcaemia and bone metastases (BOONEKAMP et al, 1986; THIÉBAUD et al, 1988; COLEMAN et al, 1988) (Fig. 1). Until recently, APD was thought to have no antitumour activity, on the evidence of two animal tumour models:

– the transplanted, osteolytic and hypercalcaemic Walker carcinosarcoma, and
– the intratibially transplanted, osteogenic and metastasising osteosarcoma.

Survival times (Kaplan plots) of rats after subcutaneous transplantation of Walker carcinoma cells, and subsequent therapy with APD and other anticancer agents are shown in Figure 2. Although APD was clearly active against hypercalcaemia in this model, survival time of the treated animals was not prolonged, and tumour growth was not inhibited in the APD groups compared to controls (KREMPIEN et al, 1988; WINGEN and SCHMÄHL, unpublished data). The lack of antitumour activity of APD and its methyl derivatives is also seen in the intratibially transplantable osteogenic osteosarcoma in rats which, as a rule, metastasises to the lungs (WINGEN et al, 1984; WINGEN and SCHMÄHL, 1985; WINGEN and WEBER, 1987; KLENNER et al, 1988b). This tumour is less chemosensitive than the Walker model, and produces large amounts of oste-

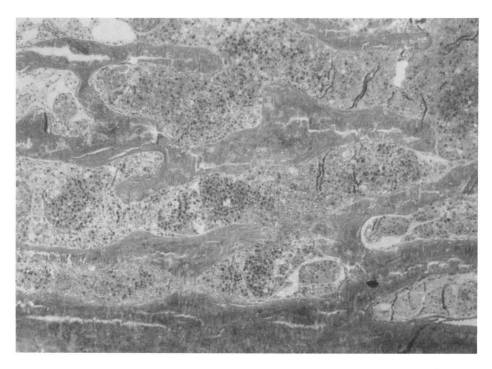

Fig. 1. Tibial trabeculae of an APD-treated rat after intratibial transplantation of 2×10^6 Walker carcinosarcoma cells. There is a lack of osteoclasts and inhibition of bone destruction even when the bone is completely surrounded by vital tumour cells.

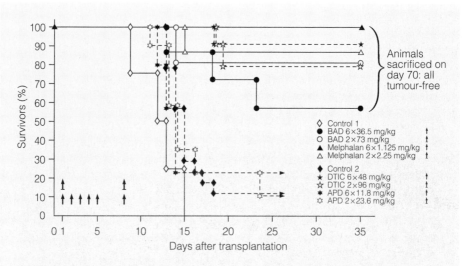

Fig. 2. Survival times (Kaplan plots) of rats with Walker carcinosarcomas, after subcutaneous transplantation of 1.5×10^6 cells on day 1, influenced by APD and other anticancer agents. Note that APD lacks antitumour efficacy even at high intravenous doses.

oid, both in the primary tumour itself and in the metastases. Autoradiography shows a high uptake of ^{14}C-APD in bone, liver and at the tumour site (Fig. 3). Nevertheless, the therapeutic efficacy of APD, even after repeated intravenous administration of high doses, is not significant (Fig. 4). As in man,

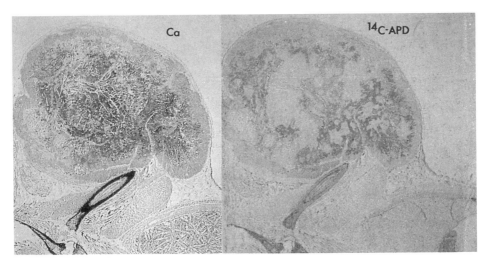

Fig. 3. A large rat osteosarcoma *(left)*, with calcium staining showing the femur and calcified areas of the tumour. On the *right* is an autoradiograph of the same area, one hour after intravenous injection of 10 mg ^{14}C-APD, showing high APD deposition in bone, liver and osteosarcoma (except in necrotic areas).

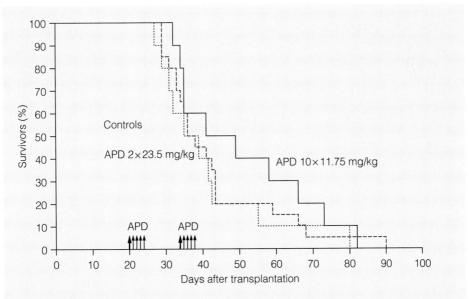

Fig. 4. Kaplan plots showing lack of significant prolongation of survival time in APD-treated osteosarcoma-bearing rats, even after high and repeated doses.

however, the survival time of these osteosarcoma-bearing rats is mainly limited by the development of pulmonary metastases, not by the growth of the primary tumour itself.

It has therefore been assumed that bisphosphonates act solely against bone metastases by inhibiting the activity of osteoclasts or precursor cells, and not by a direct action on tumour cells.

The autochthonous mammary carcinoma (AMC) model

In contrast to these findings, recent experiments – using a slow-growing autochthonous mammary carcinoma in rats induced by methylnitrosourea (BERGER et al, 1983; ZELLER and BERGER, 1984; BERGER and ZELLER, 1984) – have revealed a significant antineoplastic action on the primary tumour after intravenous and intraperitoneal APD administration (WINGEN et al, 1988). With regard to patients with bone metastases, it was thought to be important to recognise possible effects of bisphosphonates on the *primary* tumour while treating the metastases with these drugs. Our aims were to investigate this action further, and to establish possible interactions between bisphosphonates and simultaneously administered anticancer drugs. The formulae of the various drugs tested in this model, as monotherapy or in combination, are shown in Figure 5. The compound 4-[4-[bis-(2-chlor-ethyl)amino]phenyl]-1-hydroxy-

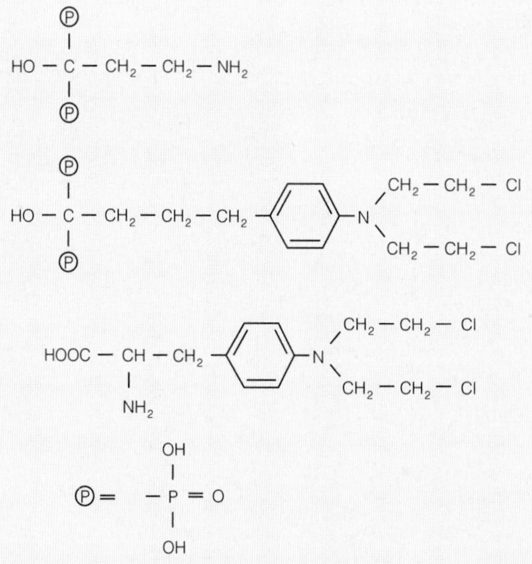

Fig. 5. Formulae of test substances used in the autochthonous mammary carcinoma model.
APD = 3-amino-1-hydroxypropylidene-1,1-bisphosphonate
BAD = 4-[4-[bis(2-chloroethyl)amino]phenyl]-1-hydroxybutane-1,1-bisphosphonate
MEL = melphalan

114

butane-1,1-bisphosphonate (BAD) was synthesised from APD and a melphalan-like anticancer agent, with the aim of combining osteotropic and anticancer activity in one molecule. Against it, we tested combinations of APD and melphalan.

Surprisingly, monotherapy with APD was found to exert a significant antitumour effect in this model, which is less chemosensitive than the transplantation models (Figs 6 and 7). An intravenous dose of 11.75 mg/kg APD daily for six weeks reduced tumour size to 5.2 cm^3, compared to 43.2 cm^3 in the placebo-treated controls (WINGEN et al, 1988). After intraperitoneal administration of the same dose for five weeks, tumour volume was 3.7 cm^3, as against 52.0 cm^3 in the control group (KLENNER et al, 1988a). A dose of 36.5 mg/kg BAD daily for four weeks was also effective, but better results were achieved with the combination of APD (11.75 mg/kg) and melphalan (0.6 mg/kg). Development of new tumours was strongly inhibited by this regimen, a result never before achieved with other drugs in this routinely used tumour model. BERGER et al (1987) demonstrated similar but weaker effects with the

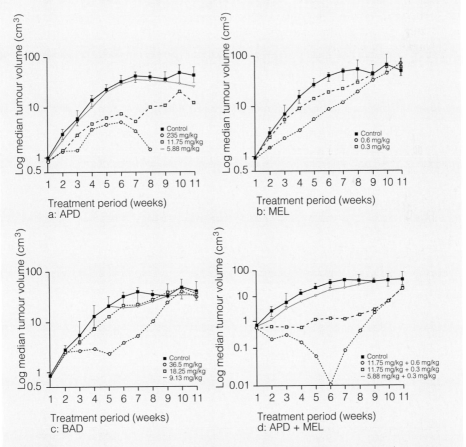

Fig. 6. The effects of various concentrations of APD, MEL, BAD, and APD and MEL in combination, on tumour growth in the autochthonous mammary carcinoma model.

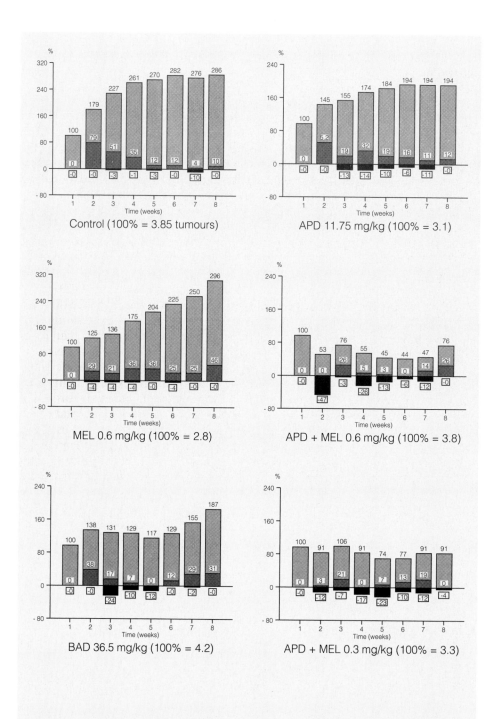

Fig. 7. Bar charts showing total numbers of tumours ▨, complete remissions ■ and tumour recurrences ■ in a control group and in groups treated with APD, BAD, MEL, and two combinations of APD and MEL. Initial numbers of tumours were calculated as 100%, differences in the following weeks being compared with the initial values.

membrane-active compound hexadecylphosphocholine, which is currently undergoing phase II studies in the treatment of the skin metastases of mammary carcinoma.

In contrast to these findings with APD and melphalan, the therapeutic actions of combined APD and tamoxifen, in six different combinations, were not additive. Indeed the mortality rate increased compared with APD treatment alone (KLENNER et al, 1988a).

The three tumour models used are summarised in Table I. The two transplantation models are characterised by a short tumour-doubling time and a relatively short survival time, whereas the autochthonous model reflects the human situation more closely.

Histological findings

To explain the discrepancies between the anticancer activity of APD in the AMC model and its lack of activity in the transplantation models, we directed our attention to the histological changes. In the AMC model, tumour cells result from several stages of malignant transformation from normal mammary gland cells. As is clear from Figure 8, the malignancy of these cells depends on tumour size and age. (These tumours appear progressively along the line of the mammary glands after tumour induction.) Small tumours contain many adenoma cells, whereas larger tumours have undergone malignant transformation to adenocarcinomas. In the experiments described above, we started treatment with APD, and combinations of APD and anticancer or anti-estrogen drugs, when the total tumour size per rat was approximately 0.8 cm^3. APD may therefore exert its anticancer activity, alone or in combination with melphalan, by inhibiting malignant transformation of the methylnitrosurea-induced adenomas.

Table I. Characteristics of the three animal models referred to in the text.

Tumour model	Doubling time (days)	Mean survival time (days)	Cause of death
Transplantable Walker carcinosarcoma	4	10–12	Primary tumour or hypercalcaemia
Transplantable osteosarcoma	10	35–40	Lung metastases
Autochthonous mammary carcinoma	19	55–60	Primary tumour or other neoplasms

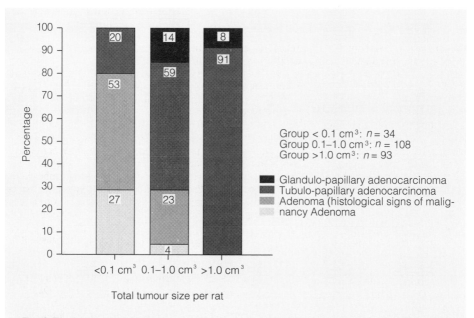

Fig. 8. The histological findings in methylnitrosourea-induced mammary carcinoma in rats, in relation to tumour size.

Conclusion

At present, the mechanism of the synergistic or supra-additive antitumour effects of APD and the alkylating agent melphalan is not understood. It is also unclear why this beneficial effect is not seen when APD is combined with the anti-estrogen tamoxifen. There are only a few references in the literature to the anticancer activity of APD and other bisphosphonates in animals (FRANCIS et al, 1980) and in humans (BIJVOET et al, 1980; MORTON et al, 1988), and no clear attempt to elucidate the possible mechanisms of action has been made. However, it now seems evident that APD has anticancer effects in addition to those on bone.

References

BERGER, M. R. and ZELLER, W. J. (1984) Wege zur rationalen präklinischen Testung antineoplatischer Chemotherapeutika. *Beitr. Onkol. 18,* 274–286.

BERGER, M., HABS, M. and SCHMÄHL, D. (1983) Noncarcinogenic chemotherapy with a combination of vincristine, methotrexate and 5-fluorouracil (VMI) in rats. *Int. J. Cancer 32,* 231–236.

BERGER, M. R., MUSCHIOL, C., SCHMÄHL, D. et al (1987) New cytostatics with experimentally different toxic profiles. *Cancer Treat. Rev. 14,* 307–317.

BIJVOET, O. L. M., FRIJLINK, W. B., JIE, K. et al (1980) APD in Paget's disease of bone. Role of the mononuclear phagocyte system? *Arthritis Rheum. 23,* 1193–1204.

BOONEKAMP, P. M., VAN DER WEE-PALS, L. J. A., VAN WIJK-VAN LENNEP, M. M. L. et al (1986) Two modes of action of bisphosphonates on osteoclastic resorption of mineralized matrix. *Bone Min. 1,* 27–39.

COLEMAN, R. E., WOLL, P. J., MILES, M. et al (1988) Treatment of bone metastases from breast cancer with (3-amino-1-hydroxypropylidene)-1,1-bisphosphonate (APD). *Br. J. Cancer 58,* 621–625.

FRANCIS, M. D., SLOUGH, C. L., BLACK, H. E. et al (1980) Diphosphonate treatment of a primary osteogenic sarcoma in a dog: a case report. *Vet. Radiol. 21,* 168.

KLENNER, T., BERGER, M. R., WINGEN, F. et al (1988a) Decreased therapeutic efficacy and increased mortality after combination treatment of 3-disodium-hydroxypropylidene-1,1-bisphosphonate (APD) and tamoxifen (TAM) in autochthonous mammary carcinoma of the rat. 13th Congress of the European Society for Medical Oncology, Lugano, Switzerland, 30 October–1 November 1988.

KLENNER, T., BLUM, H., KREMPIEN, B. et al (1988b) Protective effect of 3-disodium-hydroxypropylidene-1,1-bisphosphonate (APD) derivatives in prophylactic treatment of experimental osteolytic bone lesions and in transplantable osteosarcoma of the rat. 13th Congress of the European Society for Medical Oncology, Lugano, Switzerland, 30 October–1 November 1988.

KREMPIEN, B., WINGEN, F., EICHMANN, T. et al (1988) Protective effects of a prophylactic treatment with the bisphosphonate 3-amino-1-hydroxypropane-1,1-bisphosphonic acid on the development of tumour osteopathies in the rat: Experimental studies with the Walker carcinosarcoma 256. *Oncology 45,* 41–46.

MORTON, A. R., CANTRILL, J. A., PILLAI, G. V. et al (1988) Sclerosis of lytic bone metastases after disodium aminohydroxypropylidene bisphosphonate (APD) in patients with breast carcinoma. *Br. Med. J. 297,* 772–773.

THIÉBAUD, D., JAEGER, P., JACQUET, A. F. et al (1988) Dose-response in the treatment of hypercalcaemia of malignancy by a single infusion of the bisphosphonate AHPrBP. *J. Clin. Oncol. 6,* 762–768.

WINGEN, F. and SCHMÄHL, D. (1985) Distribution of 3-amino-1-hydroxypropane-1,1-diphosphonic acid in rats and effects on rat osteosarcoma. *Arzneimittelforsch. Drug Res. 35,* 1565–1571.

WINGEN, F. and WEBER, E. (1987) Changing metastasic patterns of a transplantable rat osteosarcoma. *Clin. Exp. Metastasis 5,* 17–26.

WINGEN, F., SCHMÄHL, D., BERGER, M. R. et al (1984) Intraosseously transplantable osteosarcoma with regularly disseminating pulmonary metastases in rats. *Cancer Lett. 23,* 201–211.

WINGEN, F., POOL, G. L., KLEIN, P. et al (1988) Anticancer activity of bisphosphonic acids in methylnitrosourea-induced mammary carcinoma of the rat – benefit of combining bisphosphonates with cytostatic agents. *Invest. New Drugs 6,* 155–167.

ZELLER, W. J. and BERGER, M. R. (1984) Chemically induced autochthonous tumour models in experimental chemotherapy. *Behring Inst. Mitt. 74,* 201–208.

Pamidronate as an adjuvant in the treatment of high-risk breast cancer – discussion paper

H. T. MOURIDSEN

Finsen Institute, Copenhagen, Denmark

A study is currently being planned in Denmark to examine the value of pamidronate (APD) as a possible adjuvant in the treatment of high-risk breast cancer. As mentioned earlier in this symposium, approximately 80% of patients with breast cancer will ultimately develop bone metastases. That was the reason why we planned this collaborative study, together with breast cancer groups in Sweden (Uppsala-Ørebro, Umeå). When planning the study several fundamental questions were discussed: the optimal duration of pamidronate therapy, and whether it should be given orally or intravenously, continuously or intermittently. At present, however, we don't know the answers.

We are using the study design shown in Figure 1. All patients in this study will receive chemotherapy – either CMF* or CEF** – randomly, and half of each group will also be randomised to pamidronate 150 mg twice daily. Pamidronate treatment is planned for four years and we plan to recruit a total of approximately 1200 patients, together with the Swedish groups.

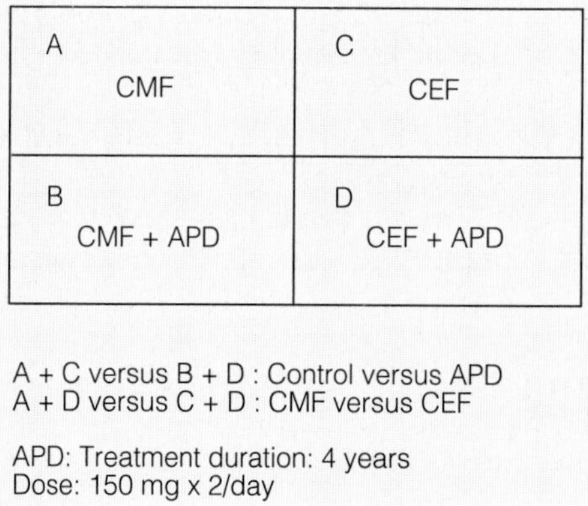

A CMF	C CEF
B CMF + APD	D CEF + APD

A + C versus B + D : Control versus APD
A + D versus C + D : CMF versus CEF

APD: Treatment duration: 4 years
Dose: 150 mg x 2/day

Fig. 1. Design of comparative study.

*CMF = cyclophosphamide/methotrexate/fluorouracil
**CEF = cyclophosphamide/epirubicin/fluorouracil

Panel discussion

Loss of bone mass

Dr C. GALLAGHER (London): Are you concerned about generalised loss of bone mass during prolonged bisphosphonate treatment, and how significant is it compared with what might be expected in this predominantly postmenopausal group?

Professor O. L. M. BIJVOET (Leiden): Over the last five or six years we have undertaken a controlled, open study of bone mass in osteoporotic patients, using 150 mg APD/day. Results show a 2.5% increase in bone mass after one year and further increases in bone mass throughout the second and third years – so at that dose there is certainly not a loss of bone but an increase. Mr Clarke's study which raised this point involved a group of patients with prostatic carcinoma, certainly not a typical population and one from which I would not draw conclusions about any long-term changes in bone mass due to APD. Remember that two Danish and two American groups have all consistently observed an increase in bone mass with bisphosphonates.

Mr N. W. CLARKE (Manchester): In our study 14 repeat tumour-free samples showed a definite decrease in bone volume and mineralisation rate at the dosage used over a six-month period.

Professor P. BURCKHARDT (Lausanne): The dose which you chose was relatively low, so it might be that the observed loss of bone is due to the underlying cancer, and has nothing to do with the effects of APD.

CLARKE: That is certainly a possibility. When the results from the control group are available we may well be able to provide an answer.

BIJVOET: You mentioned both bone mass and mineralisation rate. We expect the latter to decrease somewhat in any patient treated with bisphosphonate because bone turnover decreases. Did you also look at calcification in APD-treated patients?

CLARKE: No, but we did look at osteoid surface and osteoid volume, both of which declined. The influence of the disease itself is probably important – most of our patients have a low mineralisation rate and either a low or low normal osteoid surface in tumour-unaffected areas.

Dr S. P. PARBHOO (London): Have you any information on bone mass after APD in the premenopausal patient, as opposed to the postmenopausal patient, most of whom have already lost some of their bone mass?

Dr S. RALSTON (Edinburgh): A placebo-controlled study reported in *The Lancet* used APD (150 mg per day by mouth) to treat steroid-induced osteoporosis in a small group of men and women (pre- and post-menopausal) and found that it significantly increased bone mass – by 19.6% on average, compared with an average loss of 8.8% in the control group (REID et al, 1988).

It is important to realise that assessing trabecular bone volume is not a good way to measure bone mass, because there can be a 30% site-to-site variation in trabecular bone volume, even from the same bone on the other side of the body. I think that the problem of reduced bone mass is probably not significant.

Clinical response

Dr A. HOWELL (Manchester): Several of the studies have shown very similar responses to APD in patients with metastatic bone disease. But why don't all patients respond objectively to APD, in terms of either stable disease or partial remission? Put another way, what are the mechanisms of resistance to APD?

Professor A. L. HARRIS (Oxford): It is difficult to answer that question without a good assay. First of all you need to know what is happening in the plasma, and whether there are changes in clearance and distribution with repeated doses. Then you must determine the mechanism of hypercalcaemia in the individual patient. Patients who relapse may require a higher dose of APD to regain control, and may eventually become resistant to it. The mechanisms of resistance will be clarified by *in vitro* studies on defined cell populations.

BURCKHARDT: Resistance to APD is almost unknown in tumour-induced hypercalcaemia. I have now treated over 130 patients with this condition, and only one patient failed to respond. However, there is another aspect to resistance, due to the general impact of cancer cells on the skeleton. These cells harm bone partly via the osteoclast, but this is not necessarily the only harmful mechanism. A treatment which acts with remarkable consistency on bone resorption will not act on all aspects of metastatic bone disease.

Professor R. D. RUBENS (London): Professor Bijvoet, you wanted to add something?

BIJVOET: Yes. In patients with tumour-induced hypercalcaemia, our experience is at variance with Professor Burckhardt's: we certainly do see resistance to APD. For instance, patients with renal cancer may respond very well the first time, but during the second or third recurrence become completely resistant. Secondly, patients with hypercalcaemia due to hyperparathyroidism or parathyroid tumour are much harder to treat, partly because their bones become resistant to APD. However, it is known from *in vitro* studies of bone that if you can overcome the inhibitory effects of parathyroid hormone or osteoblast-derived factors on bone, you can also overcome their effect on APD.

Combination therapy

Dr R. HULTBORN (Gothenberg): There are at least two reports showing that combining APD with tamoxifen in animals reduces survival rates. Do you have any data on the combination in humans?

Dr A. VAN HOLTEN (Leiden): We have some data on the survival of patients with and without APD, but I must stress that both groups received variable antitumour treatment throughout. That said, there are to date no differences in overall survival, but there is a difference in skeletal disease-free interval, favouring APD. Unfortunately we do not yet have a subset analysis comparing patients on tamoxifen and APD with those receiving tamoxifen alone, so I cannot answer the specific question.

Spinal cord compression

VAN HOLTEN: There have been several references to spinal cord compression in patients treated with APD. Can you speculate on the reasons for this rather serious complication of therapy?

Dr R. COLEMAN (Edinburgh): This is a somewhat anecdotal complication. In some cases it has been due to extraosseous soft tissue extension of tumour rather than to bone. This emphasises the point that APD needs to be combined with specific anticancer therapy, otherwise the basic disease will not be treated.

Professor A. LIPTON (Hershey, USA): I agree with Dr Coleman that there is extraosseous extension into the vertebral foramina. Patients with prostatic cancer and back pain need to be investigated – by myelography or magnetic resonance imaging – for possible early spinal cord compression before they start on APD.

Intravenous dosage

Dr B. CANTWELL (Newcastle upon Tyne): What is the most rapid infusion rate for APD, bearing in mind the problems of renal toxicity that have arisen with the other bisphosphonates?

BIJVOET: The reason we infuse APD slowly is to avoid precipitation of calcium bisphosphonate complexes, which may have caused the renal damage seen in patients treated with etidronate, due to rapid infusion. After all, pharmacokinetic data show that whether you have the same amount over four hours or 24 hours is unimportant – there is 60% retention in both cases. The pharmacodynamic data which I reported in my paper suggest that patients may require further treatment with APD after 3–4 weeks without therapy. Regarding dose equivalence, I believe that 90 mg APD intravenously over four weeks is equivalent to 300 mg orally daily. These are not precise data but working figures.

Reference

REID, I. R., KING, A. R., ALEXANDER, C. J. et al (1988) Prevention of steroid-induced osteoporosis with (3-amino-1-hydroxypropylidene)-1,1-bisphosphonate (APD). Lancet i, 143–146.